THE EMOTIONALLY DISTURBED CHILD
An Inquiry into Family Patterns

J. LOUISE DESPERT, M.D., is former Associate Professor of Clinical Psychiatry, Cornell University Medical College, and Associate Attending Psychiatrist, Payne Whitney Psychiatric Clinic, New York Hospital. She is widely known as a teacher and consultant in the child psychiatry field, in which her studies have ranged from personality development in normal children to severe personality deviations in child schizophrenia. Dr. Despert is a member of the American Medical Association, a Fellow of the American Psychiatric Association, a charter member of the American Academy of Child Psychiatry, and affiliated with other professional organizations. Her previous books include the popular *Children of Divorce* (Doubleday Dolphin Books) and *Schizophrenia in Childhood: Collected Papers* (Brunner, 1968).

THE EMOTIONALLY DISTURBED CHILD

An Inquiry into Family Patterns

J. LOUISE DESPERT, M.D.

Formerly
THE EMOTIONALLY DISTURBED
CHILD—THEN AND NOW

Anchor Books
Doubleday & Company, Inc.
Garden City, New York

This book was originally published as *The Emotionally Disturbed Child—Then and Now* by Robert Brunner, Inc., in 1965. The Anchor Books edition is published by arrangement with Robert Brunner, Inc.

Anchor Books edition: 1970

ACKNOWLEDGMENTS

The author gratefully acknowledges permission to quote from the sources named.

To the *American Journal of Orthopsychiatry* for "Some Considerations Relating to the Genesis of Autistic Behavior in Children" by J. Louise Despert.

To Grune & Stratton, Inc., New York, for the quotation from "The Differential Diagnosis Between Obsessive-Compulsive Neurosis and Schizophrenia in Children" by J. Louise Despert which appeared in *Psychopathology of Childhood* edited by P. Hoch and J. Zubin, 1955. To the *American Journal of Psychiatry* for the case report quoted in "Psychopathology of Stuttering" by J. Louise Despert.

FOREWORD

In my first approach to this subject, *The Emotionally Disturbed Child*, I visualized the conventional clinical account of emotional illness in children. We are familiar with it. In doing research, however, for the topic's historical background I was at once impressed with the fact that prior to the mid-nineteenth century no evidence could be found of emotional illness in children as we understand it today. To fix the beginning at this level is actually being generous, since the latter part of the nineteenth century offers only indirect episodic tales of abuses of children, leaving it to the imagination of the reader to project attending emotional ills. It was tempting to go further back. But where? How? Surely, through the centuries children have been reared in families, have matured into men, and they must have had anxieties and frustrations. Of these, unfortunately, there seems to be no record. Thus I was inveigled to pore over manuscripts, manuscripts which at first seemed to have little or no connection with childhood emotional ills. Even at the end of this search it cannot be said that I have become very much enlightened, and the impression thus would be that emotional disturbance in the child is properly a twentieth century phenomenon. Timeless and universal it must of necessity have been, even if we cannot back up the assumption. We cannot, however, minimize the fact that even under the short span of time under consideration, i.e., the first half of the twentieth century, there has been a progression in incidence.

Not only have facilities been created at a rapid pace for psychotherapy of children. But we must look further: we know, for instance, that one out of sixteen in the general population will be or has been in treatment at a state hospital, to mention only this type of psychotherapy. In the ranks of the state hospitals' population are many patients with emotional ills which have long gone undetected and untreated. The acute psychotic episode of the adult has its beginnings long before adulthood. We may well ask why, if there are so many "happy" children, are there so many unhappy and emotionally disturbed adults?

In the pages of this book I have attempted to give a picture of emotional disturbance in children and its background of family maladjustment. This is not an all-inclusive survey of emotional illness in children, rather, a sampling, also an inquiry and a raising of questions as to the how and why of emotional illness in children.

J.L.D.

CONTENTS

INTRODUCTION

The long-forgotten child is coming into his own. It is frequently said of the twentieth century that it is the century of the child. It has also been said that it is the age of anxiety (W. H. Auden,[1] Rollo May,[2] Paul Tillich[3]). There is more than a coincidence in the apposition of these two generalities. That the attention increasingly lavished on the child has not brought him all the blessings that could be expected of the vast interest and intense preoccupation—this deserves careful scrutiny.

Is the child today really happier? Is he making a better adjustment to life? Is he (both as child and adult) less vulnerable to pernicious mass influences? Is he better prepared to meet adult responsibilities?

We have only partial answers to these questions. Perhaps at this time the latter can be answered only by further questioning. Why, for instance, are emotional disturbances and maladjustments of both child and adult on the increase? The figures confront us. We may try to circumvent them by pleading greater awareness. Greater awareness there is, but is it totally determining? So is greater availability of psychiatric resources claimed. But are the clinical facilities not increased as the need for them becomes greater? According to a 1951 Public Health Report by Pennell[4] there were (during 1950) 1,228 mental health clinics in operation in the United States, at least 902 serving children. An estimated minimum of 150,000 child patients were seen there during the year 1950. These figures can hardly be considered to represent a maximum, since checking on all clinics does not bring out total response. Additional facts escape statistical computation completely: it is well known that all children who should receive treatment do not, as clinic waiting lists will attest. Furthermore, the figures given in this report do not include children treated in private practice, well-child clinics, pediatric clinics (the latter two officially given over to preventive care, but functioning as well in the capacity of therapeutic centers), or private psychiatric clinics. Nor are special schools, special hospitals receiving children in need of residential care, considered in this report.

Some of the gaps are filled in by Morse's and Limburg's report.[5] According to them, 485 known psychiatric outpatient clinics (travelling as well as stationary) were operating in the United States and territories in 1947. Figures are hazy about the total number of patients treated there, and in particular the number of children. A conservative estimate of 100,000 children for the year 1947 can be given. Even though the figures may not cover identical categories, the reader will not fail to spot the rapid increase denoted by the 1947-1950 reports.

Incomplete as these figures may be, they tell a story with a meaning that we cannot afford to disregard or misinterpret. The high incidence of divorce, the increase of psychoses (child and adult) and the number of suicides, the increase in juvenile delinquency—these are indications that all is not well in our understanding and approach to the child, that our methods of fostering normal emotional growth are inadequate or misdirected.

The child has become an object of fond (?) attention from the educator, the pediatrician, the legalist, the psychologist, the psychiatrist, the minister—all in a matter of half a century. Not so closely related but of significance is the growing class of creators of entertainment devised for the child's special benefit: theatre, music, television shows, etc.

There are many signs of the rapid evolution from oblivion to limelight, perhaps none more significant than the one embodied in the very terminology used. The concept of the "emotionally disturbed child" is of recent import. While its exact appearance in the literature cannot be pinpointed, a conservative estimate would place it at a little more than a quarter of a century ago, when its present-day meaning was crystallized. Nothing can better reflect our change of attitude toward emotional disturbance in children than a cursory examination of the terms used to describe deviations in child behavior. Children have been been considered in turn "possessed . . . wicked . . . guilty . . . insubordinate." When they came to be called "problem children"—a kindly euphemism—the indication was that they were at least given some attention.

Through the centuries, outside of a few bright spots such as the Greek society, the child was hardly considered a specific entity of the human order. Even these bright spots are not so impressive in the light of our knowledge of modern psychology. Time-honored educational methods, while perhaps more enlightened, were nonetheless insensitive. Of insight into the inner life of the child there was none.

It was only during the sixteenth century that pediatrics books appeared, denoting for the first time an awareness of differences between the child and the adult. Medical men realized at last that a child is not a small edition of his adult counterpart, and that his physical care and treatment require a departure from the long-accepted ways. So much for his body. But what of his feelings, his aspirations, his frustrations? Of these intangibles no record can be found, with rare exceptions, until the nineteenth century.

The child's position in the average family of the masses was for centuries roughly in this order: father, cattle, mother, child. He was part of the chattel and in certain societies could be sold. The Roman Code hovered over the legislature of most European countries until recent times with little alteration. Its influence, waning and somewhat humanized, is still perceived in the family structure of early American Colonial life.

In its initial and most rigid expression the Roman Code showed little sympathy for the child. The Law of the Twelve Tables granted the father the right to sell his child, and it clearly specified that the thing sold was the right of the buyer to make use of, as extensively as he would, the physical and intellectual potentialities of the child.

The tasks demanded of him well into the nineteenth century were so disproportionate with his status and stature as a child that one wonders how such feats of physical endurance could be accomplished. Witness the laws written at the end of the nineteenth century to put a stop to some of the existing abuses and *limit* the number of children employed at night. Difficult as it is to recreate in one's mind the physical hardships, it is even more of a challenge to envision the inner feelings of the stunted young beings at work. Some contemporaneous writings are tragically eloquent on this subject. The work of man was lightened by the Industrial Revolution, even though this may not have been its primary purpose, but the child was unquestionably the loser in this wave of progress.

Even in the privileged classes the child failed to be privileged. His education was handed down rather indiscriminately, the child eventually ending with a low type of servant, not a highly selected tutor or preceptor. Modern psychologists are prone to put the Victorian era under fire. But that a child could at least be seen, if not heard, is evidence of a gain in recognition, since, indeed, prior to that period he was relegated to oblivion, and not even seen.

One must reach the twentieth century to see the dawn of an awareness of the child's inner life, his emotional needs, and his emotional problems. Leo Kanner has rightly pointed out that child psychiatry could not have existed before the twentieth century.[6]

In the concept of the emotionally disturbed child there is an understanding and compassion which only the twentieth century could have fostered. Perhaps some of our attitudes toward children are better understood in terms of the long neglect and ignorance of the child's plight through the centuries. Some of the psychological problems which will be considered in the following pages are in part related to these attitudes.

Part One

WHAT PRICE LOVE?—A STORY

The Oblers are settling down in their quarters for a peaceful evening. Ma Obler marches out of the kitchen first with David in tow, and it won't be long before Pa, having cleared the dishes, joins them.

This is a daily ritual, and one might as well say a symbol. A symbol of their family life, and one which will want elaboration.

Pa has now joined them, and the settling down is not altogether for a peaceful evening, what with deafening noises and the tension in the air. Sprawled on the sofa bed full-length with his knees slightly raised, David is obviously enjoying the blaring music and the frantic shooting of some Western movie he has been awaiting eagerly. Ma sits in an easy chair close to his head with her everlasting sock-mending, looking up at intervals toward the screen which is directly in front of them both. From time to time David stretches out, reaches for his mother's bare arm, touches it lightly with an incongruous bleat: "Ma."

As for Pa, it takes some hard looking to discover him on the far side of the living room, quietly smoking his pipe and craning his neck to steal a side glimpse of the movie in which fortunately he is not too interested. He is a slight man and sinks deep in the arm chair. His pipe jutting out at a belligerent angle asserts the man.

If I have selected the Oblers out of a large stock of clinical material, and just-plain-human material seen through the clinical eye, it is because their story brings out nuances about the essence of maternal love. In a book on legal and emotional divorce, *Children of Divorce*,[1] I presented, under the heading "Love Is Enough," the Lewis family as an ideal milieu for the rearing of children. Benjie, adopted into this warm, united, and harmonious family group—joys, frustrations, and all—flowered into a well-integrated, normally aggressive youngster, intellectually functioning to his capacity, outgoing, fond of people and well-liked by them.

The Oblers' station in life is somewhat similar to that of the Lewises. However, their story is in sharp contrast with the Lewis story. For several years they have been working as a couple—caretaker and housekeeper—for a lawyer whose professional activities keep him in a nearby town.

Martin Snell, a widower and childless, is overburdened with the demands of his heavy practice. After his wife's death he had a fling at running his house, *his* way. This was before the Obler regime. Gradually, he has faded into the recurring shadow of a weekend guest, the paying kind. Bills outstanding and mechanical breakdowns in urgent need of a solution await him with the unfailing regularity of nightfall.

Although Burt's unprepossessing appearance should have precluded such initiative on his part, Martin Snell made it his business at first to give orders and suggestions to him rather than to Kate. Brilliant attorney though he is, no point could be argued when the woman was about. The moment he would approach Burt to communicate his intentions, there Kate would be, snorting,

"You think he understood what you told him? Well, he didn't, the dope! You'd better tell me and I'll see to it that it's done."

Strange as it may seem, Burt, who had heretofore listened to him with a bright enough expression, suddenly appeared the perfect moron, his mind a blank. Unwilling to meddle with their personal relationship and weary at the very thought of having to run the estate by remote control, Martin Snell had given up. The whole affair was humiliating, and he wanted to forget the man's wan smile and the faint shrug of his shoulders as he turned to his wife for orders. His private name for Burt after this was "the slave." Like many another slave, Burt carried his role with a self-effacement and a dignity that should put to shame the most hardened slave-driver.

The estate, maintained by the Oblers with the aid of an occasional hired hand, is in fact run by Kate. A wing of the main house is set aside for the help. The way Kate Obler has utilized these quarters tells us something more about the emotional climate of this family. Two bedrooms are on the second floor, while the room on the ground floor is, technically, a living room. When shown her quarters, Kate flatly announced that the two bedrooms would be for herself and her son David; Pa Obler would have to sleep downstairs. Pa, tagging along with his small staccato step, gave his acquiescence by merely nodding. It mattered not that the living room had only a narrow couch. If Ma said he was to sleep there, so he would.

The owner had been somewhat puzzled by what seemed an extravagant request—three bedrooms for a working couple. The motivation behind the apparent extravagance became clear to him in no time at all. Ma Obler simply could not part from David, nor would she tolerate her husband nearby for reasons which will become obvious as we get better acquainted with this family.

As for Mr. Snell, of necessity he soon became acquainted with Kate's domineering personality. This meant a gradual succession of compromises on his part. Why all the compromises? Well, Kate has solid qualities as an organizer. And if her organizing is at times on a tangent, even at cross purposes, with his own wishes, on the other hand she can be relied upon to do a thorough job and at all times hold the fort as if it were her own fortress. If the Oblers were to stay—and Mr. Snell wanted them to stay, especially Burt—compromises there had to be.

Not that the lawyer is able completely to overlook all the possessive mannerisms of his housekeeper. He still winces at the sound of "my living room . . . my garden . . . my basement . . . my freezer . . . my garage . . . ," and similar figures of speech applied to his possessions. "All forever mine"— this is Kate Obler taking over.

Shortly after their arrival, and without warning, she had

replaced the ancient brocade table runner of his living room with a flowery throw rug of her own making.

This he protested. "I know everything here tends to become yours. But this piece, no . . . no. Shabby though it may be at present, my wife designed it, and I insist on its remaining right here."

In recounting the episode to his friends, the lawyer, who is not without a sense of humor, usually adds, "Well, I'm grateful that my bedroom is not included, not yet. That would be a little confusing. . . . Yes, she stops there, one wonders why. . . . And on the whole I am safe. I'm holding on to the deeds."

In the face of small details, significant as they may be, one should not hasten to conclude that Kate Obler is a selfish, grabbing woman. On the contrary, she is the epitome of devotion and kindness—if one may so interpret her feelings—and is full to the brim of good will toward her fellow man. To the exclusion of her husband, of course: for him no honeyed words, no spontaneous offer of assistance. Indeed, she almost begrudges him the minimum of sympathy expected to flow between marriage partners, however indifferent they may be toward one another.

Not long before they came to their job at Mr. Snell's, Burt had been gravely ill, and in the course of a long stay at the hospital had undergone a major operation. The medical bills, a drain on their meager resources, were settled in small monthly payments to the last cent. But how had Kate resolved the resentment that this great loss from the common fund aroused in her? By simple accounting. Month after month she matched dollar for dollar until the same amount spent on Burt's surgery was available for a trip she had long coveted: a visit to her aged father, who had earlier returned to his place of birth in the Old World. She felt doubly justified in this leveling expenditure, since she might never see her father again, while David hardly knew him at all. Needless to say David was going along.

To all but her husband, Kate is ready to do a good turn. Let her hear of a young couple in the village unable to attend a social function because no one is available to tend the baby, and Kate is on the phone offering her services as a baby sitter. Untrained but experienced, home nursing is her particular avocation; and no family need fear lack of care if Kate, whose ears are sensitive to grapevine information, can pick up the news.

Kate Obler is an attractive, plump woman, somewhat overpowering, in her early sixties. A cheerful one, always smiling, often singing, she never seems to lose sight of her avowed life purpose—helping people. She is frightfully busy thinking and carrying out ways of doing something for someone. Indeed, her recurring explanation for any enterprise is, "I like to help."

Like Benjie's mother, Kate Obler has had what could be considered by many of us a hard life. The eldest of six children, she lost her mother early, and automatically was called upon to bring up her siblings, acting as a substitute for their mother.

Her father's favorite, and very close to him from the first, she developed an excessive attachment to him. The father never remarried. Struggling with a tool factory so small you could call it a one-man tool factory (and should that even be called a factory?), he spent long hours in his shop. Thus, Kate was to her brothers and sisters the sum total of parental influence. A loving big sister she was, but an exacting one. She was exacting for herself and did not spare others. She developed all the domestic skills; she was heir to the maintenance of the house as well, and learned after a manner to tighten bolts, fix house gadgets, replace washers, tinker with electrical wiring, and perform other such manly activities.

The fact that electricity becomes in her hands a deadly weapon does not deter her from attempting to improve installations made by licensed electricians. Will she let years of experience under the guidance of a first-class mechanic, her father, be wasted on her? The blowouts and breakdowns which invariably follow in the wake of her non-licensed enterprises only reveal to her some hidden defect, engineered and overlooked by the licensed operator. In Kate's eyes, the problem is simply one of delayed reaction. And fortunate it is that the defect should come to light at just this time, for who knows what catastrophe might have been in the making? So does Kate elucidate the mystery of ever-recurring short circuits, stalling pumps, and recalcitrant furnaces.

Irrepressible Kate, who since her early adolescence has been the indispensable moving power in the house—mother to her siblings then; man and woman all in one, then and now.

With such a background it is not surprising that Kate Obler married rather late. How she came to marry, and why she married Burt, she explains in simple terms. She had a strong desire to have children of her own. Under the conditions of her life in a small Southern town, with drudgery every day and little outside contact, marrying was no easy matter.

Burt Obler, a Northerner by birth, had moved with his family to the South while still a child. Now in his middle sixties, he works on the lawyer's estate as caretaker, and is officially in charge. Although he is about the same height as his wife, he appears smaller. He is a hard-working man who seems to plunge into manual work as an escape from some inner turmoils. Yet he is quite capable of completely relaxing, almost falling apart, after a day of exhaustive labor. He says little, and one gets the impression that he never ceases to look for reassurance that his job is well done, that he is approved of. With his employer as with his wife, he tries to ingratiate himself by offering to do little things that are not demanded of him. He has gone through a fairly long life, insecure, yet not beaten. His proud carriage is witness that he has not given up, even though, as we shall see, his lot has not been the most fortunate either.

The complete financial failure of his father had thrown the family into a destitute situation when he was eight years old. Since then, Burt has seen furniture go out because the last installments were not paid; he has often been on the edge of starvation, and living has been a matter of survival by any and all devices possible. Of the nine children in the family he seems to have been the one most able to cope with the odds so unmercifully piled up against them. He felt at one with his kin through all their sufferings, until the opportunity came to enlist in the army. Then, without warning, he enlisted.

The army suited him well. He was relieved of financial worries, and he liked the order and regimentation. He looked up to his superiors as omnipotent and all-knowing; even as he climbed to a sergeant's rank, power was never a lure to him. Nor did he assert himself when he made his home with Kate; and it can be safely assumed that his passivity was the *leitmotiv* of their married life.

From the start, marriage has been for Burt a tough assignment. Try as he would, he was not able to meet Kate's demands. Not that they seemed excessive to him, since a wife has claims on her husband. But it was the way she went at him, without respite: by plain, outright nagging. She was devoted to him to be sure, seeing fussily to his clothes and his food, suggesting that he invite this friend more often and that one less or none at all; and this for his own good, not for any benefit she might derive through her own counsel. All this he fully appreciated.

During the course of their marriage, his relation to Kate has altered considerably. In the beginning, her charm and beauty, her proud poise, had made her seem nearly unattainable in his eyes, and free from any flaw. Gradually, she had revealed herself as anything but flawless. Hoping for an eventual serenity that never came, he had given in at every turn. However, far from mollifying her, his compliance only increased her irritation. His often-said "Yes, darling," at first mellowed with tenderness, came to sound more and more like the smart "Yes, sir!" of the private first-class standing at attention before his drill sergeant. The "Yes, darling" shot in the air so fast that it often fell dramatically out of context in a situation that called for a denial with no alternative.

He became more submissive, less loving. In a slow progression he withdrew into a shell. He would be found smoking his pipe for longer and longer periods, lost in his thoughts. It was odd, he reflected, that he should in the long run pattern himself after his father, whose taciturnity and moody spells had so often blocked him in his attempts at confiding. Lonely in his family, he had later found much to share with his colleagues in the army. But now in his own home lonely feelings were upon him again.

He was puzzled too, though not troubled, by Kate's sudden radiance and glow of happiness whenever "The Girls" were visiting or when she was returning from one of her weekly dates with them. He wished that she could be a little more discreet or controlled when he appeared on the scene and her face visibly dropped with discontent. Again and again he rationalized that he was not envious of her friends and, on the contrary, was pleased to see anew the sparkle in her eyes and the animation of her whole personality, so reminiscent of courtship-time. Were these precious moments irretrievably lost to him? Was he at fault in not having nurtured and tendered them? And if so, how had it happened?

"The Girls" had been an institution with Kate almost as long as he had known her. A club leader . . . she had always been interested in political, social, and other issues close to the heart of civic-minded women. Even in her native village, with all her house chores and family responsibilities, she had managed to set aside a few hours weekly to sew and chat with "The Girls." In the several army posts she and Burt had known since their marriage, she had invariably succeeded in collecting a sampling of women for her weekly get-togethers. He had been satisfied to putter silently backstage preparing drinks, since this usually brought a word of thanks from Kate —enough to sustain him for a little while.

These ruminations Burt does not communicate to anyone. They remain in his own private world.

If he says little of personal matters, Kate is more fluent. To almost anyone within hearing distance Kate tells of her long suffering as a wife. She sees herself withering in her life with Burt. "I'm ambitious and I'll get someplace," she still vows, even though getting someplace at the Oblers' age would be a rather remarkable feat. True, as an army wife she has "gone places," but not in the way she would have liked. All her married life she has deplored her husband's lack of ambition, his lack of drive. He has been satisfied with the uneventful security of his never-failing monthly paycheck. This she has resented, although for a long time she would not push him to leave the army. She had not quite dared, at least for some years.

The end of his military career came all too soon for Burt. It was Kate's suggestion—and he had promptly endorsed it— that the modest capital they had amassed in the army should be invested in the purchase of a farm. The venture proved a disastrous miscalculation. A series of jobs followed, each appearing to Kate, the incorrigible optimist, as more promising than the last, but ending in no better way. These were jobs requiring teamwork, and the Oblers could never achieve the unity of purpose that makes for successful teamwork. At odds with each other, how could they be of one mind on their job?

To hear Kate, Burt has been a very attractive man. "Attractive to other women," she readily adds. It would be difficult to judge the question at this time, although Burt Obler retains a certain almost adolescent quality and a candid blue-eyed expression which is refreshing to behold. His erect body carriage, the stamp of his stints in the army, also belies his years.

Kate's story is that her husband has not been faithful to her. When, early in their marriage, they were stationed in the Philippines, she drifted away from him because of his alleged affair with a Filipino girl. Fleeting suspicions also gnawed at her about his relations with other army wives. Later, when they came back to her home town, she was positive that he had taken up with a Negro girl and was supporting her financially. To the casual eye Burt Obler does not look the part. But some wives see their husbands in a special light. They think their men have attributes irresistible to women at large. This is Kate's given reason for her indifference to her husband's sexual approaches. It would also explain the crack in their marriage, although she does not acknowledge an outright failure or crack, since she sees herself as a great cementing force. In her occasional outbursts of resentment, and by way of justification for banishing him from her bedroom, she will be heard exploding, "I hate him! I hate him!"

With so much hostility generated, with so much tension stirring about, why have these two beings not lived as separates, and indeed gone further and actually separated? Why? The unavoidable answer is that they cannot, because they need each other in their neurotic marriage ties. It is to her husband's philandering—actual or fantasied—that Kate attributes her strong negative feelings toward him. But were there not danger signals already present before their marriage? She chose him and he chose her. The choice was not mere accident, even though neither of them may recognize the basis for their choice.

When, on leave from the army, Burt came to propose to Kate, he had already known her in their little village for several years. He was powerfully attracted by her will to dominate and control, a will which he needed, unbeknownst to himself. And so it was with Kate, who had seen this man's possibilities. She loved him for qualities which essentially are not an integral part of a virile personality. He was tender, thoughtful, attentive to subtle changes in her mood. Of virile qualities she wanted none.

Her inarticulate antagonism toward men reveals itself in an episode that she often tells with undisguised mirth. Their engagement was to be announced, and he had come resplendent in his uniform, laden with flowers and presents. He stood shyly before her as she opened the door. At that solemn moment she did not look the radiant fiancée he had expected. Playfully, so she claims, she had shouted to her dog, "Sic the damned Yankee!"

Of course it was only a joke. How revealing a joke! Her underlying hostility toward men was breaking through, but Kate would be nonplussed if such an interpretation were tendered to her.

At the end of his leave they were married, and she started with him for his post in the Philippines. She felt lonely and even estranged from her husband. With time, she thought, she would outgrow the feeling of estrangement. He was so much at ease in this exotic background! Perhaps he would eventually draw her into the social life he seemed so familiar with. Yet there was something wrong, but she could not give it a name. Here was a young man she had long known in her village. She had anticipated life with him in a design free from complications—creating a home and having him fit into it. But she now found it difficult to speak his language, to accept his gestures of love. She busied herself with innumerable chores, drifting further and further away from her home. She learned many of the ways of the natives, building a canoe entirely of her own design and making. Being gregarious, she also engaged in a multiplicity of minor social activities which consumed much of her time.

12

"The Girls" were a boon to her through the difficult times, and she lived for the carefree, playful hours she had with them. It seemed unbelievable—and not a little disturbing—that their company could make her feel so warm, so young again; whereas Burt need only appear to get her bristling with hatred.

It was obvious that the breach between herself and her husband was widening. Explosions followed periods of mute, accumulated tension. After several years she decided to "go back home." Then and there a marriage-pattern was set which recurred almost with the regularity of a pendulum: after she had spent some time at her father's home, her husband would come, plead with her, and take her back. They have been married now close to thirty-five years, and the first half of this span of time was spent seesaw-fashion, with Kate moving between her father's and her husband's homes.

The Oblers were a childless couple. Then the incredible happened. During a period of reconciliation, she became pregnant. David was born.

In that instant Kate Obler was completely metamorphosed. She now had a purpose. It mattered little or not to her whether Burt was faithful, since her rejection of him was now complete and irrevocable. They continued to live under the same roof. Ma Obler, was, as the saying goes, wrapped up in her child. But it would be more accurate to say that she wrapped herself completely around him. It does not take much knowledge of psychology to forecast the emotional struggle the child would eventually have to go through to free himself. And to date he has not done so.

Kate likes to linger over the early years when her friends alluded to the "Madonna and child," a picture she willingly portrayed for them. She also likes to linger over David's post-infancy years, recalling them as the happiest time of her own life. The two of them would start out for long days in the woods. "Make yourself beautiful, Mommy," David would insist when she neglected her make-up. Dressed in bright cottons, humming a gay tune, a picnic basket on her arm, she would lead the way, David trotting on his small legs a few paces behind her. Those were days of enchanted intimacy. Through his mother's eyes David saw the fluttering of vari-colored insects amid rich, dense foliage. From these days he

13

has retained the ability to perceive through all his senses the multitudinous themes of the forest. From these days she has retained, besides her glorious memories, two distinctive habits: one being to call her husband by her son's name more frequently than by his own; and the other to dress—or rather undress—herself in very brief, colorful shorts and halter at the least provocation, such for example as working in the garden. To her employer's dismay she sees no incongruity in greeting his guests at the door this way, an elderly housekeeper in tropical play clothes.

This is Kate, child of Nature, center of her world, constrained by no rules of ethics but her own. Her world tightly encloses her son, the beloved; and never were the bonds between them closer than they were back in the forest during the day-long outings. That was her work of creation, initiating the boy to the sounds, the images, and the rhythms of tropical Nature. When the family eventually came back to her own home ground, these early impressions were to be the golden standard of her later experiences.

Whenever something goes awry, Kate—having plunged headlong into some erratic enterprise, and on from this into a crisis—invariably retorts to her employer, "We do everything to please you." And, in all sincerity, she does. However, it would not occur to her to inquire into his preferences, so certain is she of knowing, perhaps better than he does, what should bring him pleasure or what is good for him. No power can stem the tide of Kate's tyrannical benevolence. And of this benevolence David, needless to say, has been from birth the chief beneficiary.

She never ceased to teach and mold her young son in ways she defined for herself as the right ways. Kate Obler always had very strong feelings about "right ways," and was determined to implant them in her son. And she always had a passion to give shape and direction to young lives, whether they were human, animal, or even belonging to the realm of plants.

One look at Kate planting, uprooting, replanting, and it appears that her passion is tantamount to a compulsion. "I like it. . . . I would like to pull weeds and make room for the flowers. And if the flowers don't make out so well, out they go. Nothing satisfies me quite so much as pulling weeds.

14

. . . I know my husband doesn't like me to come near the flower beds, but in the end he appreciates the weeding."

The garden is her kingdom. There her rule is absolute. If she decides that "it's cheaper to buy radishes and onions than grow them," out they go, and her employer, generally articulate enough, fails to convince her that these vegetables have been thriving under her predecessor's care. Once, in the heat of a discussion where her opinion was challenged, she impulsively exploded, "I'm always right!" This slip she retrieved with some difficulty. It was not at all what she had meant, and she was at a loss to explain such a slip of the tongue. Nevertheless, only a profound conviction that she cannot falter in her judgment would explain her authoritative ways.

David from the start complied with the rules and even enjoyed the world created around him by his mother's loving obsession. There was endless fun in the games she taught him. If he did not miss the companionship of other children, it was only because he had absolutely none of it. His mother was the beginning and the end of all his emotional experiences. She spared him the frustrations and disappointments attending the business of growing up. She would always anticipate his most tenuous wishes. He lived in a fool's paradise. The payoff was to come along with the demands of compulsory education.

Meanwhile, he was living in a closed world, a world closed particularly to Burt, who was now like a stranger in his own home. Rather feebly, Kate attempted once to make the separation complete, but decided that "after all, the boy needs a father," and stayed on.

Surely a boy needs a father. But what sort of a father had David? What could it be when subtly—and not too subtly—the mother was infusing in the child's mind an image of his father not likely to help him identify with a male adult? The hostility and contempt she had for her man were voiced in front of the child as well as to Burt directly.

Today we see the aftermath of her handiwork. Should his father make such a slip as anyone might, David is apt to turn to the company and, by way of jocular explanation, say—with a screwing motion of his finger at his temple—"Well, you know my old man!"

It is not only that Ma Obler is disparaging of her husband. Her son-worship also tends to annihilate all extraneous influences. One solid block, two interlocking units—one will. The remainder is a background to be molded and disciplined toward her foremost purpose, that of making David happy. For instance, it would never occur to her to prepare anything but David's favorite dishes. Far from hiding this fact, she places a dish on her employer's table with the accompanying statement, full of maternal pride, "David likes it."

Martin Snell, whose tastes do not always coincide with David's, attacks his roast glumly and with pangs of guilt. He feels that he owes it to his housekeeper to enjoy her culinary efforts. But at intervals the words, like the food, stick in his throat. Would he ever forget the day she had greeted him with the cheery news that a wonderful creamy dessert was awaiting him? She had made it especially for David. Now, David, erratic in his preferences, did not want it. It was offered so warmly and with such an aura of exclusiveness that he had remained dumbfounded. He could not, however, bring himself to do honors to the very special masterpiece. Said Kate, "Never mind if you are not hungry this noon. It will keep till tonight." It did, and Mr. Snell, now weakening, ate the much-lauded dessert.

Kate's gift for putting his possessions to David's use has brought no end of surprise to the lawyer. One day, walking idly from lawn to garden, he came upon a strange sight on his tennis court: on one side of the net just in front of the retaining wall was a mound—bale of hay piled upon bale of hay—and all crowned with a sheet of tar paper. He found Kate unruffled by the news of his discovery. "David wants to do a little target practice . . . bows and arrows. . . . It won't do any harm to the court, and it's safe with a wall at the back of the target. . . . But never you fear, that will pass. . . . Don't you remember the raft on the pond? He has given that up. And the gun target? Didn't he remove it after a few days? . . . Just you give him at most two or three weeks, and he'll be fed up with this too."

The world is David's oyster. His mother sees to that.

Trouble really began for David when he entered school. An intelligent boy, he found it extremely difficult to concentrate

on the subjects taught there. They were of no interest to him, and were due to remain so for a long time. He was constantly drifting into vague, dreamy images which had nothing to do with the three R's. The boys and girls in his home town seemed to find it palatable to sit and liste[...]
Not he. Again and again he was reprimand[...]
ing attention." He came home weeping to [...]
have preferred to keep him under her wi[...]
David, so sensitive, so carefully nurtured. [...]
for what she considered the struggle with [...]
there, in the sanctuary of the school, she [...]
and could not protect him.

Any child of pre-school age is bound [...]
anxieties. These early years are the pho[...]
and real or fantasied animals hold mild [...]
of normal emotional growth. But with D[...]
considerably beyond the normal range. [...]
quently awakened by his nightmares. S[...]
with her, little inconvenience was caused [...]
simply reach out and cuddle him. With th[...]
attendance his nightmares increased in n[...]
For the first time she became worried a[...]
with the nightly panics. She turned to th[...]
assured her that in time the boy would outgrow his fears. He held the same view regarding the child's temper tantrums.

The boy had learned at the usual age all the motor skills, sitting, walking, playing ball, and so forth. But Kate was puzzled that, in contrast, he did not talk until very late and with a halting that gradually developed into a frank stutter. With unlimited patience and determination she taught him to speak slowly in short sentences. David, who was always so compliant with her, would not, or could not, heed her suggestions. She sensed defeat, and this was very distasteful to her.

There was also this matter of wetting the bed. Was this the bright, gentle, and docile youngster she thought she had made of David? Frustrated and unbelieving, she was left completely helpless. She coaxed, threatened, promised rewards, punished, all to no avail.

As time went on he began to grimace—in technical terminology he developed facial tics—which brought her to a pitch of exasperation.

Now eighteen, David is far from being a normally adjusted boy. He is at least two years behind in his studies, although of good intelligence. His facial tics and stutter are still with him. He is shy and almost friendless. Girls are a closed book to him, a fact which, incidentally, does not displease his mother. "He has time for that. He's just a baby."

The most malignant sign is the behavior which has substituted for his early temper tantrums: when faced with a difficult task he is prone to become tense, irritable, and explosive. Unable to cope with his inner feelings, he soon finds himself in a kind of panic which causes him to lose control, break any object at hand, and run—literally run—out of the house. He has no insight into the nature and the violence of his impulses at such moments, but he is very much frightened by that very violence.

Psychologists are familiar with the surge of these unconscious forces. An adolescent boy who has not freed himself from his mother, whose inner core is so weak, so tense, so immature, experiences guilt and anxiety-feelings which must explode in some way.

Hard as it is to believe, Kate still calls her son, "Baby," and "Pussycat." The boy enjoys and fiercely resents his mother's blind devotion to him. He may tease her for it, he may be embarrassed before strangers, but he basks in it too.

He also liberally uses his mother's ever-present readiness to come to his rescue, however ludicrous the end result may be. Recently, having registered for the military reserve (he wants to graduate from high school, which will take him another two years), he was asked to go to the county seat and be fingerprinted. A major enterprise for him, although barely a fifteen mile bus trip. He was planning to make it on his own, as would be suitable for an aspiring warrior. At the last moment he lost his nerve and asked Ma to go with him. "Only don't call me Pussycat before the recruiting non-com," was his manly request. The possibility that his father might accompany him never entered David's mind. Presenting himself at the recruiting center, he was told to go to the police station. So, off to the police station went Ma and David, a

18

strange couple wandering about wide-eyed, asking their way to the fingerprinting outfit.

What does the future hold for David? We are fully aware that he has built up a distorted image of marriage relationships. He sees his parents in constant bickering, and often steps in with a soothing word for his father or his mother. When his father is grateful, his mother takes the word as a personal offense, and is furious. On the other hand, David seldom needs to be actively on his mother's side, since Burt is the swallowing kind.

In their joint employment Burt officially is in charge. But is he really? David sees his mother outlining in offendingly minute detail the daily schedule of the man-in-charge. Repeatedly he hears her criticizing the way the man-in-charge works, but taking credit for all ultimate good results, since the planning was hers anyway. He is aware of his father's meek requests for money, parsimoniously handed out to him for haircuts or cigarettes. Their employer can be amused at her devastating thoroughness, humorously calling her "Boss Lady." To David this is no laughing matter. He has often wondered why his mother is so hard on the old fellow. She must have been in love with him once, but even traces of that he has not witnessed. He has only known bitterness and hostility one way, abject submission the other way.

Granted, his father has allowed him all the guns he could buy—even bought him one himself, with Mother's approval, to be sure. David spends hours oiling, polishing, cleaning his collection, but would his old man pick up a gun and go hunting with him? No. Why? Why is he so easily satisfied, the day's labor over, to put on slippers and sit almost motionless in his corner until bed time? What sort of a man was he before he married? Perhaps very different than he is today. Perhaps more manly. Would his mother somehow be responsible for his soft behavior? David does not want to go too deeply into these disturbing questions. On the whole, they remain unanswered.

When in a family the roles of man and woman are so obviously reversed, only confusion and anxiety can result for the children.

On the face of it, love has not been lacking for David. His

19

mother has indulged him in every possible way. She is cease-lessly preoccupied with his welfare and his happiness, as she sees them. And she has been known to rise to his defense with the fierce instinct of a tigress protecting her cub, when the slightest criticism of his achievements was made, for in-stance at school. If David does not get the highest marks it is obviously the teacher's fault. He tries his best, and she knows that his best should be enough to satisfy any teacher. Up to school she trots to set the teacher right when the injus-tice seems gross enough to her.

The over-indulgence has softened David. And incongruous it is to see this nearly six-foot-tall, muscular and well-developed boy so spineless in an emotional sense.

Let us be mindful that Benjie was not spared any of those hardships his family suffered. Rather, he was asked to share them, accepting them for the warp and woof of daily living as the rest of the family did. We have seen that Benjie was none the worse for it. Indeed, his mother, ever-giving in her selfless way, supported him in his growth to boyhood and, at this date, young manhood. This she had done for the older children as well.

Mrs. Obler gives, and she gives a great deal. But is her gift comparable to that of Benjie's mother? If anything it is over-whelming, so there is no question of deficiency. What we are dealing with here is a quality of love rather than a magni-tude. It should be immediately obvious that we have before us two very different kinds of love.

In contrast to the richness and plenitude of the love life of Benjie's mother, Mrs. Obler's marriage has been anything but gratifying. Could it be otherwise, seeing that she entered her marriage with confused and ambivalent feelings toward the man she was to marry? Was she not enduringly her father's darling, identifying with him and taking into the marriage partnership a very masculine role? We will agree that she has given generously of herself, but *what* has she given?

When built on the foundation of frustrated marital love, what is maternal love but a type of short-changing? And so it is that David has been getting, not his due, but credit owing to his father. The love of a mother can foster emotional growth and it can also smother it. The latter has been David's experience.

While the story of David may appear in spots as somewhat extreme, it is by no means a rare story. Many of the emotionally disturbed children entering a psychiatrist's office present variations of the Obler theme. The shadings may be subtler; or they may also be more gross, and the outcome more devastating.

David is at present still protected by his family—in essence, by his mother. The time must come when he will have to go it alone. The eventuality of marriage is not far off. And even before that he must think of preparing himself as a wage earner. How will he stand the test of demands made by life at the adult level?

He plans to join the army as his father did. Is he, like his father, passively to accept army regulations and become, if not a shining recruit, at least a very acceptable member of the armed forces? Or, in the face of frustrations which he is not prepared to accept and which are bound to come his way, is he likely to explode? We can expect the latter. Military authority and paternal authority are clearly alike, and we know what contempt paternal authority inspires in David.

Girls have not had any attraction for him, because his mother stands heavily in the way. Loving a girl could only give him guilt feelings which would throw him off his fragile emotional balance.

There are signs that David is on the verge of revolting against his mother's tyrannical love, although this does not mean that he is coincidentally shedding his morbid dependence upon her. "He's getting fresh," moans his mother, when he snaps at her instead of "yes-mother"-ing her.

There was a violent—and most unusual—scene between them recently. Kate wants him to become a mechanic like her father, and the army has appealed to her from the start as a place for him because of the facilities for specialized training it offers to those who enlist. David now has become impatient to tinker with a car; and one day he put an ultimatum to his mother about buying an old jalopy that he could pull apart and, with luck, put together again. This would

21

require his invading the one free garage-space, and, therefore, first having to secure Mr. Snell's permission.

"Ask him yourself," suggested his mother. However, for moral support she stood by as David put his strange request to the lawyer.

"Couldn't you learn at one of the repair shops in the village?" inquired Mr. Snell. "You make yourself useful in small ways, somebody will take an interest in you and teach you the tricks."

Little did he know David's aversion for entering a new situation. No, there was no chance, the boy was sure, even though he had not given it a try. But Mr. Snell remained firm in his refusal. The space was needed for his guests.

Grasping at last the finality of the decision, David turned viciously on his mother. "How do you expect me to become a mechanic if I can't even tinker with an old car?" His face distorted with rage, his voice mounting to a swell of exasperation, he let go a volley of insults at Kate, who for some moments remained silent.

Then she rose to his defense. "He's ambitious, like me. Don't fret, Baby. Another year and I'll buy you a car, your own car. I promise you that." This is how Kate resolves for her boy the threat of frustration—through additional yielding.

Whichever way you look at David's emotional adjustment, the cards are stacked against him. At this stage he could be helped, were his mother to develop an awareness of the boy's plight and a willingness to relinquish her managing.

Shortly after the outburst about the garage, Mrs. Obler turned to her employer. Did he know someone who could give her a "consultation" about David? Were there not people to whom one could turn for advice? On television she had seen children who were being treated by some specialist for troubles very much like his. A very peculiar way of treating them, she reckoned—with words and games. But it seemed to work.

There was a traveling clinic once a week at the county seat, he told her, and the guidance teacher at school should be able to give her information regarding its services.

Her first interview at the clinic proved a complete fiasco. She want to see her husband for? He had no part in the mat-

22

ter. And if anything were to be accomplished, it would only be through her. If they could not tell her how to do it, there was no need for future discussion. It was the shortest interview the social worker had ever had with a client. Out marched Kate, her head high, in an aura of righteousness and enlightenment which was to be with her for some time.

Such an outcome the lawyer could easily have predicted. He had seen Kate's glassy look when he attempts to put across directions about the way he would like her to do some work. The attentive tilt of her head would seem to indicate her eagerness to learn her employer's intentions, but the curtain has come down. Though the sounds are quite distinct, the meaning of words is lost on her. The unconscious block is total.

Kate has an uncanny ability to shut out unwelcome experience completely. This imperviousness protects not only herself but also David, who, at eighteen, still hangs on to the magical wishful thinking of early childhood. She has already resolved that there is nothing the matter with David, only the short-lived bad humor of teen-agers. No doubt it is a good healthy sign that he doesn't resign himself to defeat as easily as his father. She will try to be more constructive in helping him realize his wishes and ambitions.

Thus ends the story of David as it stands to date. However, for him it is only the beginning of an emotionally crippled life.

Part Two

THE LONG-FORGOTTEN CHILD

The term "emotionally disturbed child" is a recent import in psychological and psychiatric literature. It crept in as a slight departure from a term previously used, "maladjusted children." In 1921 a paper appeared which brought out that the emotionally maladjusted, of all groups of maladjusted children, had received the least attention.[1] So far as can be ascertained it was not until 1925 that the term "emotionally disturbed" was defined as it now stands, curiously enough in causative relation to skin diseases.[2] However, from material available, it appears that it was not applied specifically to children until 1932, in an article by Sullivan.[3] The prestige of Menninger was instrumental in the wide recognition given this concept when it was officially incorporated into the classifications of veterans with emotional disturbances.[4]

As applied to the child, the concept of emotional disturbance does not go back over a quarter of a century. In a very short span of time the expression has become a household word, due largely to radio and television spreading knowledge of mental disturbances. Today Johnny's minor aberrations of behavior are brushed off as indications that he is "emotionally upset," or "emotionally disturbed."

This term does not stand for new forms of mental illness, and new symptoms have not cropped up under its wing. It represents an evolution of our attitudes toward the mentally ill. Children affected with what we would describe today as neurotic and psychotic illness were variously labelled through the ages as "possessed," "wicked," "guilty," "insubordinate," "incorrigible," "unstable," "maladjusted," and "problem-children," roughly in this order. Close as they are to us, the last three epithets do not reveal any empathy for the child. Rather they put on him the onus of guilt and the accusation of his having failed society. Embodied in the more modern view are an insight and compassion which have long been lacking.

Attempting to trace the history of emotional illness as it concerns the child, or at least what would correspond to emotional illness in terms of present knowledge, one is baffled to find that records begin no further back than the twentieth century. Indeed, Kanner could write,

When the twentieth century made its first appearance there was not—and there could not be—anything that might in any sense be regarded as child psychiatry.[5]

Any student of human behavior will have noted that writings on child psychiatry do not reach beyond the line of demarcation set by Kanner, if and when they concern themselves with historical background. Undoubtedly, children had experienced emotional disturbances before the twentieth century. Though they would not be described in modern terminology, it should be possible to single out and identify symptoms equivalent to what we observe today. Zilboorg and Henry, in a work of erudition, have pushed the frontiers back to the sixteenth century with accounts of rare instances of mental illness in children from that time on to the nineteenth century.[6] More will be said about the rarities when these periods of time are considered.

Looking further back into the historical past, one encounters additional hindrances. In order to try to reconstruct emotional disease in children, one must plunge into the chronicles of the time—writings on education, philosophy, and history—only to come up with very little knowledge of the child's emotional status. This may appear a very unorthodox way to investigate the subject. But how else could it be done when pertinent documents are not available?[7]

Take, for instance, an exhaustive study of the French people's life from its origin to the end of the eighteenth century.[8] It distinguishes itself for the omission of material pertaining to children. There is a great deal about family living, food, dress, and social and religious activities, but children are not mentioned except for a few passing references to their eating habits. One chapter deals with religious and official holidays, such as Easter, with the blessing of eggs and the various rejoicings associated with the festival. At length there are described exchanges of gifts between parents, neighbors, and friends. But the children do not appear. The kind of omission met here is not specific to this work; other writings of the time are just as reticent.

Consequently, one is at a loss to project the life of children in the family, let alone their emotional problems. One can of course go to such archives as report on the life of historical figures such as Joan of Arc, and find many homey details about her growing years in her family—a reconstruction made necessary at the time of her trial. How would it hold the mirror to the life of contemporary children? Nevertheless, the absence of the child in chronicles which propose to reflect the life of the times cannot be other than meaningful.

This brings to mind an apt comment made by a scholarly librarian at the *Bibliothèque Nationale,* Paris. When approached for help in the search for data about children during the Middle Ages, she exclaimed, *"Mais c'est un travail de Romain!* . . . Perhaps if you read the daily chronicles of monks and nuns you might gather a few, very few items. . . ."* Her unfinished sentence left a forbidding trail of unknowns. This is quoted as an indication of the gigantic undertaking a search of this order would represent.

Consider that, prior to the sixteenth century, the child from a medical point of view was not differentiated from the adult. The first three pediatrics texts[9] appeared in England in 1545 (*The Boke On Children,* by Thomas Phayre), in Spain in 1551 (*Libro del Regimiento de la Salud y de las Enfermedades de los Niños,* by Lobera de Avila), and lastly in

France in 1565 (*De la Manière de Gouverner les Enfants dès leur Naissance*, by Simon de Vallambert). In passing, note the "governing" of children from birth on. It is indeed revealing of the despotic attitudes of the past toward children and in striking contrast with present-day liberalism.

Even as these books on pediatrics appeared in the sixteenth century, there was a lag in customs, and we find a famous physician from the period of Louis XIV (1643-1715), Dr. Gui Patin,[10] prescribing that a three-month-old child be bled twice for a head cold. Other physicians of the period seem to have been even more radical, one having bled a three-day-old baby suffering from erysipelas.

That much for the child's body. But what of his feelings, his aspirations, his frustrations? Of these intangibles, records cannot be found. It will be necessary to search here and there in writings not directly pertaining to children in the attempt to build a picture of the child's emotional vicissitudes through the centuries.

Here is a splendid opportunity for research, though a painstaking and perhaps not too rewarding enterprise: to ascertain the emotional status of the child in family and society through the centuries.

While awaiting this research, one can stop and reflect upon the significance of the long tradition of oblivion and of the vacuum evidenced in historical records. One can consider this meaning in the light of otherwise known historical facts such as the high infant and child mortality of centuries past. One can see as responsible not only such physical agents as epidemics and malnutrition, but also emotional factors inherent in the neglect of and disinterest in children. Other well-known historical facts such as the children's crusades deserve to be examined in the same emotional context.

Surely our attitudes toward children today are related to and determined by attitudes in the past. Why has no one dared go back beyond the twentieth century? Is it that the heartlessness and cruelty toward children which peer through related subjects as found in historical documents have proved unbearable to the modern student of behavior?

In the following pages we will get glimpses, however fleeting, of the way the family and society treated and mistreated the child. Of his emotional adjustments and maladjustments little can be learned. This study does not propose to be exhaustive, nor is it claimed that the samplings given are consistently representative. Our goals are limited; and if the curiosity of the reader is aroused, that is sufficient reward.

CHILDREN OF THE BIBLE

The emergence of children's figures through the reading of the Bible is laden with complexity. Consider that the child's life was offered up in religious rituals; and while the sufferings and the great sacrifice of the parents are also portrayed, the cruelty to the child is laid out as an undeniable fact. Witness the story of the hundred-year-old Abraham and his two sons.

> And Sarah saw the son of Hagar the Egyptian, which she had born unto Abraham, mocking.
> Wherefore she said unto Abraham, "Cast out this bondwoman and her son; for the son of this bondwoman shall not be heir with my son."[11]

First, Abraham casts out Hagar and her child, with the child left under the bushes in danger of death, though later saved by God. (Genesis xxi. 9, 10). Further, Abraham complies with God's order to sacrifice his then only son, Isaac (Genesis xxii. 1, 2), who was also saved.

Take also Elijah, mocked by the children and dealing with them as we find in the second Book of Kings ii. 24):

> And he turned back, and looked on them, and cursed them in the name of the Lord. And there came forth two she bears out of the wood, and tare forty and two children of them.

The Bible is replete with examples of cruelty to children, although they are not always of such magnitude as that found in Herod's order to sacrifice all children.[12]

> Then Herod, when he saw that he was mocked of the wise men, was exceeding wroth, and sent forth, and slew all the children that were in Bethlehem, and in all the coasts thereof, from two years old and under, according to the time which he had diligently inquired of the wise men.

Cruelty to the human child as seen in the sacrifices was carried on through the ages and took on a renewed intensity during the medieval period.

Children also seem to have been expected to carry out functions and chores considerably beyond their years, a characteristic which is found through later periods, such as the Middle Ages, and to a lesser degree through the nineteenth century. "Manasseh was twelve years old when he began to reign."[13] "Josiah was eight years old when he began to reign."[14] At twelve years Jesus is depicted as "taking up God's work" in the very adult way of the doctors of the temple.[15]

But more essentially one is impressed with the arbitrariness in selecting the children, either for sacrifice or for elevated positions. Consider Nebuchadnezzar, commanding

> the master of his eunuchs that he should bring certain of the children of Israel, and of the king's seed, and of the princes; Children in whom was no blemish, but well favoured, and skillful in all wisdom, and cunning in knowledge, and understanding science, and such as had ability to stand in the king's palace. . . .[16]

However incomplete a picture these few scattered illustrations may help to build, we are nevertheless impressed with the utter contempt for the child as an individual. No participation is demanded of him; he is simply disposed of at the will of his elders. While writings of a given period cannot be taken to give a complete and faithful reflection of the customs of a society during that period, they do give some conception of what the general emotional tone might have been.

33

SOME IMPRESSIONS OF THE CHILD
AMONG THE HEBREWS

It would take a Hebrew scholar to ferret out evidence of the emotional life of the child from the vast Hebrew literature which concerns itself with religious beliefs, education, history of the people, and so forth.

Early education was given in the home, with young children being taught the Hebrew alphabet.[17] Children were asked to read the Pentateuch, starting with Leviticus. Thus they became acquainted with the Laws. Long passages from the Bible were memorized as soon as the child was able to speak. He was also taught very early to translate Hebrew into Aramaic, which was the language commonly used. Beginning with the study of the Bible at a very early age, higher education continued with a more exhaustive study of the Bible, to which gymnastics, singing, thorough acquaintance with the hygienic laws, and "esoteric knowledge" were added.

In their approach to formal education the Hebrews show an awareness of individual differences. It is more a matter of intellectual differences than emotional differences, but at least the individual is given some consideration. We learn that pupils were classified into four types: pupils swift to hear and swift to lose (in remembering), pupils slow to hear and slow to lose, pupils swift to hear and slow to lose ("a happy lot"), pupils slow to hear and swift to lose ("an evil lot"). A similar classification was expressed in terms of sponge, funnel, strainer, and sieve.

There is further indication that deficient students were given additional attention, either by the teacher or by those students who were more proficient. Great attention was paid to the texts from which the students were to study. "When you teach your son, teach him out of a corrected book." The teacher was encouraged to be outwardly strict but inwardly a friendly counsellor. "Push them (students) away with the left hand and draw them near with your right."

While the women were superficially treated as inferior to men—not permitted to be witnesses or judges, exempt from reading the Torah, kept in separate galleries in the temple, and not allowed polygamy, which was permitted to men only—we are told that they were, as mothers, equal to the fathers in the eyes of their children. The intellectual and moral education of the boys was automatically entrusted to groups of men (temple), and, as a consequence, the education of the daughters was of greater concern to the parents. Women were held down to homemaking activities. Married women never worked in the fields. In contrast to education in Greek and Roman societies, religion was a very important factor.

We gain no knowledge of the child's emotional life, but we are aware that the family presents a picture of a unified group with the roles of man and woman clearly defined and strong moral principles in force.

ANCIENT GREECE

In considering ancient Greece two types of civilization will be touched upon: Spartan and Athenian.

Sparta. The core of society under Spartan rule was military awareness and preparation. Thus developed a rigid social state with all things subordinated to government needs.[18] In the middle of the ninth century B.C., Lycurgus formulated a code of law which established a military state and defined a military education that was to be long in use. In the words of Aristotle (384-321 B.C.), "Sparta prepared and trained for war and in peace rusted like a sword in its scabbard."[19]

The newborn child was examined, and it was decided by a council of elders whether he was strong enough to live and serve the military state. If he was too weak he was exposed.[20] Figures are not available on the actual number or relative proportion of children who were victims of this form of infanticide. Historians are at variance regarding this moot point. Goodsell for instance writes,

> Exposure was sanctioned by law, but was probably not so frequent as some writers would have us think. More commonly this fate was reserved for girls and for illegitimate children, although boys were sometimes exposed by poor parents to escape the burden of rearing them, and by well-

to-do parents to avoid too minute a division of the family property.[21]

But Cubberly presents the problem more bluntly: "if it (the newborn) did not appear to be a promising child, it was exposed to die in the mountains."[22] There is no indication that the baby was eased into death through some humane form of euthanasia, and the plain fact is that he was abandoned to be destroyed, probably by wild animals, while "alive and kicking."

About the feelings of all parties concerned—that is, the parents, and in particular the mother—we find no trace outside of poetry and the drama. But maternal love has existed through the ages, and it takes little ingenuity to reconstruct the anxiety of the mother during pregnancy and at the time of delivery, when she anticipated the possibility of the barbarian destruction of her child. Surely there was a carryover in her relationship to her remaining children, the ones who had been allowed to live.

Infanticide in this and other forms was to plague succeeding societies well into the seventeenth and eighteenth centuries.

In Sparta, if the infant was considered fit he was formally adopted by the state but left in the care of his mother until he was seven. Swaddling was not permitted, since it was thought to interfere with physical growth. Left alone in the dark, he was not permitted to scream so that he might from the outset become tough and develop self-control. The means used to prevent the screaming are not defined, but it can be safely assumed that considerable anxiety arose in the child from the rejection of his need for comfort.

The boy's training began when he reached seven. From seven to eighteen he lived in public barracks where he was taught the well-defined Spartan ideals and expected to conform to Spartan conduct. The boys were classified into three age groups, with older and stronger ones in care of the younger. It was a frankly military organization with no trace of feminine influence. Training was severe, with food deliberately limited in quantity. The boy in training was permitted to forage, but was whipped if caught. Thus it was hoped he would learn to become crafty for the necessities of wartime. He was lightly clothed and went barefoot in winter. He slept without covering on his straw pallet, switching at fifteen to a bed of rushes.

Physical hardship constituted an ideal. It was important to become tough through physical drill, running, leaping, boxing, wrestling and fighting. If music was allowed, it was in its military form to help marching. Competition was at its highest. The ultimate goal was to win by any means; biting and even gouging were considered lawful, and even encouraged. Dancing as "patriotic and religious inspiration" was taught.

But of intellectual education there was little. The Laws of Lycurgus and a few selections from Homer were sufficient achievements. Listening to the conversation of older men was considered a means of gaining knowledge. This passive receptiveness of the young before their elders as a means of imbibing knowledge and wisdom was to thrive for centuries to come. Moral training seems to have been achieved through companionship with an older man who was set as a model.

Girls remained at home, but received much the same education as boys. Gymnastics were included in their training with a view towards making them strong for child bearing. Dancing and singing were practiced, and certain religious festivals made it possible for the girls to join the boys in celebration.

Education for the Spartan child, and particularly the boys, was conspicuously lacking in intellectual and artistic goals. As to emotions, we get a very rudimentary pattern of characteristics considered ideal by the society—characteristics thought to be virile, though only adolescent. Although the Spartan boy was considered a man at thirty and compelled to marry, it is noteworthy that he continued to live in the public barracks and could visit his wife only "clandestinely." In terms of present-day psychology, emotional development did not go beyond an immature, homosexual level. I am not referring here to the overt practice of homosexuality, although this must, of necessity, have also thrived in the face of conditions described.

Athens. In Athens, which became a democracy in 510-508 B.C., an early education very similar to that of Sparta was sponsored. Training for service to the state was also the aim. But there was a fundamental difference in that the Athenian citizen was trained for peace rather than for war. The man with a well-rounded education was considered most useful to the state. Training was for citizenship, and a richer education was thought to be beneficial for citizenship. The Athenian, in contrast to the Spartan, had ample opportunity for cultural training and broader character development.

In Athens the infant did not escape the fate of the new-born of Sparta. He was also examined at birth; not by state representatives, however, but by his father. If he was thought unfit, he was exposed. Judging from Graves' account, a certain subtlety of purpose creeps into the motivation for selecting the infants to be exposed.

> While the newly born were often exposed, this was because the father, rather than the state, felt that the child would not be a credit to him, or that his family was already large enough.[23]

As considerations of the family as a whole and of the father's feelings toward his offspring, these are evidence of a timid incursion into personal responsibility and choice.

Again, figures are unavailable. But very possibly, since the motivation was not so sweeping, exposure was less frequent than in the case of Sparta.

Unlike her Spartan counterpart, the Athenian mother was fully entrusted with the charge of her child, boy or girl, until the age of seven. The Greeks, both Athenians and Spartans, failed, however, to recognize the right of any mother to the child she had borne, since even in Athens the care of the child fell almost invariably to slaves. Socially inferior to their husbands, poorly trained, transferring their duties to slaves, the women had little influence over their children.

Perhaps more than the Greek writings, their art has given us accurate and vivid pictures of the child's life in his family. A volume compiled by Anita E. Klein some twenty years ago presents a selection of Greek art works related to the life of the child from birth to adolescence.[24] Mothers and slave nurses are depicted as warm and loving, but it is clear that they were also capable of inflicting severe physical punishment. A number of art works represent children pleading for leniency or "tugging violently in hope of escaping the ordeal." A choice method of punishment was hitting the child with a sandal. Other plates depict the readily discernible whip marks on a child's body.

The children appear healthy, cheerful, often active in a game—perhaps too uniformly so—with no stamp of individual character. The ingenuity and multiplicity of games and toys devised for the young attest to interest in the child's needs for motor expression and enjoyment. The child is also shown playing with domestic animals and riding horses; and there are realistic details which bring out the time-honored sadistic attitudes of children toward animals.

The close tie to the slave nurse is reflected in pictures of graves with inscriptions to beloved old nurses. Representations of school activities done in terra cotta are common. The total picture is one of great contrast to the life of the Spartan child.

The girl in the Athenian home led a very restricted life and was instructed only in household duties. While there may have been scant opportunity for identification with the mother, the slave from the point of view of warmth was probably a fair substitute for the mother figure.

At seven the boy was sent to school in the care of a slave. The slave, usually unfit for any other duty because of age and/or physical disability, had complete charge, nonetheless, of the boy and of his moral education and could whip him whenever he saw fit. Wisdom in his handling of the child, if it were there, must have depended on chance or parental selection, not on the training or qualifications of the slave as an educator.

According to some historians, the educational pattern was not only different from that of Sparta, but also in some respects inferior to it.

It would seem from this entrusting of the child to the moral care of slaves, such as the nurse and pedagogue, that

Athens, while broader than Sparta in its training, was less strict about habit formation in early life. . . . In the rights of women and in habit formation among children, Athens was excelled by Sparta; but upon the whole, the Athenian education was far superior to the Spartan in allowing more opportunity for individual development.[25]

In his early years the boy actually attended two schools, one for music and literature, the other for gymnastics. We see here the beginnings of compulsory education—at least for boys—since the state required that as a minimum reading, writing, music, and gymnastics be taught.

Without going through the historical developments which determined the growth of individualism and personal freedom, let us note a fact commented upon by some historians, in particular Graves. Some change in this direction must have taken place, if we take literally the biting observations of Aristophanes (444-380 B.C.):

It would seem that children became impudent, cunning, and impure; wives turned shrewish, extravagant, and unfaithful; husbands neglected their duties as householders and citizens in a search for disreputable and dishonest gain; slaves became disobedient, lazy, and disloyal; skepticism and license were rampant, and confusion was general. It was individualism run riot.[26]

The Sophists, while influencing the education of adolescents, had probably very little influence on the very young child. Pythagoras (580-500 B.C.) formulated a socialist system which attempted to achieve integration between the individual and society.

Because of their influence on education, three philosophers, Socrates (470-399 B.C.), Plato (427-347 B.C.), and Aristotle (384-321 B.C.) claim our attention. In his dialectical approach Socrates stimulated reasoning by the question-and-answer method. Plato describes his ideal in *The Republic*. We are far from the state as defined by the Spartans, but in his plan of family life much of the concept of control is enhanced. The family unit as such is lost in favor of the larger structure of the state. The military goals and the severe discipline of the Spartans, however, are lacking. Women and men, moreover, are to be considered equal and to receive special training.

Betterment of the race and measures for improved breeding are included in his plan. In his ideal state, control means the dissolving of the family as a structure: children and parents are not to know each other, but all men are to act as fathers to all children. Prevention of intermarriage between brothers and sisters is to be achieved through a careful check and recording of births. Women are considered fit to bear children from twenty to forty, men fertile from twenty-five to fifty-five.

Again, as in Sparta, children are to be selected by the state, and exposed if found unfit. If healthy, they are to be reared in a state nursery by mothers and mother-substitutes (nurses). Breast feeding is to be only for a short period, possibly to prevent deep attachments in the child-mother relationship. There is an attempt carefully to control topics and forms suitable for children, as seen in the works of imagination selected for the young. In contrast to the Spartan scheme, the ideal is "subordination of the body to the spirit."

> The two arts of music and gymnastics are not really designed, the one for the training of the soul, the other for the training of the body, but the teachers of both have in view chiefly the improvement of the soul. (*Republic*, III, 40).

Although the primary purpose of education was not training for war, Plato, nevertheless, advocated that children be "spectators of war," so that as future soldiers they might become more proficient.

We are assured by Graves that "*The Republic* had practically no immediate effect upon education or any other institution of Athens."[26]

In his *Politics* Aristotle expresses views on the education of children from birth to adolescence. The subordination of instinctual impulses to rational behavior through growth and education, and the process of sublimation, as it is known in present-day terminology, are glimpsed in a formulation such as the following.

42

As the body is prior in order of generation to the soul, so the irrational is prior to the rational. The proof is that anger, will, and desire are implanted in children from their very birth: but reason and understanding are developed as they grow older. (*Politics*, VII 15.)

Exposing is still condoned, and a rudimentary form of eugenics is considered. Abortion as a means of reducing the size of the family is approved.

One notes the high moralistic tone of the meticulous and somewhat rigid educational rules: what games should be encouraged, what stories should be told and what language used, etc. On the other hand, he encourages the spontaneous play of young children as foreign to the adults who are all too eager to direct the young in their play.

Formal schooling extended from the ages of seven to twenty-one. These fifteen years were divided into two periods by puberty. Intellectual, musical, and artistic pursuits were encouraged. Aesthetic enjoyment was recognized and fostered as part of the art and musical study. Women, being considered inferior to men, received only a limited education.

Aristotle's philosophy was to play a continued role through the Renaissance and Reformation periods.

Although Greek civilization is, relatively speaking, a bright spot in the life-story of the child through the ages, it can be seen from the preceding pages that even then the child did not fare so well. He was recognized in the abstract as man in the process of growth, requiring special approaches to facilitate and improve the growth process. Nevertheless, he was subjected to mighty forces outside of his family which nullified the tender personal devotion that individual loving parents might afford.

To begin with, he had to be granted the very right to live through powerful agents, the state or paternal authority. It matters little whether exposure was only episodic or very frequent, since the issue is one of principle rather than magnitude. He apparently did not know his mother in the close, warm, personal child-mother relationship which makes for security. Even if the mother-son relation had been permitted to be close and personal, surely the threat to the mother's offspring as embodied in the custom of exposure must have played a significant role in her attitude toward her living children. After one child had been destroyed she might develop toward the next child a defensive detachment or, on the contrary, an excessive devotion and preoccupation. We have no way of knowing; we can only assume. What is certain is that the child as a being unto himself received very little consideration.

ANCIENT ROME

The Roman family is generally described as the "patriarchal family" par excellence. It represents the emergence of the family as it is, with some variations, known to date. The family was regarded as sacred, and the father was all-powerful. It was more a religious than a social organization, for the ancestors were the protecting gods of their descendants, in divine form *Manes* and *Lares*. The Roman father had the right to reject his child at birth, but infanticide is thought to have been not so widely practiced as it was in Greece.[27]

The father's *patria potestas* was absolute and extended well into the adulthood of the son's and the daughter's married lives. He had the right of life and death over his children. He might "scourge his children, sell them into slavery, banish them from the country, or put them to death."[28] Beauvallet points out that the father did not have actually the right to kill his child as a father, but only as a judge.

> The numerous examples which are recounted in the Latin literature of cases where the father used this right (life and death) show us that the *pater familias* acted less as a private individual than as a magistrate and, as it were, by virtue of a tacit transfer of public power. (My transl.)[29]

There is evidence in Seneca (3 B.C.-A.D. 65) that the father would turn to several members of the family in the moments of his decision, so that the power of life and death over persons (wife and children) who were under his domination was somewhat attenuated.

It is specified that when the son was sold as a slave he could not stay in Rome, but was to be sent into enemy territory.[30] The son was introduced to the rites and traditions of the ancestor cult in preparation for the time when his father would die. The relegation of the rest of the family, including the mother, to a minor role is in evidence. We see it in the son's initiation by his father into the religious traditions, and in the exclusion of the mother when dramatic situations arose which involved her child. "Even in cases of divorce, the children remain with their father."[31]

Some historians take great pain to stress that the *patria potestas* was an instrument used by the father in the interest of the family and the city. The right of the father to destroy his child, however, whether as a father or as a representative of the law, remained unchallenged. Sometimes the father used his right in an attenuated form, less destructively but punitively. *Abdicatio* was the right of the father to chase the "guilty son" out of his house. There is no indication of what would become of the son, but there emerges here a manner of dealing with delinquency which became more and more popular as the centuries went on. The rejection of the offspring, whether he was sold as a slave or chased out of the house, was an extension into time of the right of destruction at birth.

It was the Law of the Twelve Tables which granted the father the right to sell his child. It was specified that the buyer was acquiring not so much the child *in toto,* but the right to make full use of his physical and intellectual activity.

This right to sell which is granted the *pater familias* is the outcome of the primitive identification of the child with the other possessions which compose the patrimony. (My transl.)[32]

Plain to see, the child was his father's property, and centuries would pass before a human quality was restored to him. It is

46

interesting to note that this same law, anticipating the possibility of shameless speculation in children, specified that, if the father were not satisfied with two successive sales, he would lose all rights and privileges conferred by the status of the *pater familias*.

Apparently the right to destroy or cast away children led to abuses. We find that Constantine I (A.D. 280?-A.D. 337), the fifth Christian Roman emperor, put pressure upon the treasury to give financial help to parents who were too poor to bring up their children. Also at this time, adoption by those parents who wanted children was initiated. Adoption papers were signed before the local bishop, and constituted a transfer of absolute power to the adoptive parent. At no time subsequently could the natural parents claim the child.

Care and education of the child in Rome mark an advance over those of Greece. To begin with, he was not turned over to slaves, and every Roman mother was expected to nurse and bring up her own child.[33] The boy was kept near his mother until the age of six or seven, at which time he became his father's shadow. In the lower classes he might be at the farm or shop. In the upper classes he trained for a military, legal, or political life, receiving instructions from his father or some older man. Meanwhile, the girl stayed at home with her mother to acquire a domestic and moral education.

In the home, reading and writing were learned through hard-driven memory work and a manner of sing-song chant which must have been hardy. Indeed, we hear echoes of it through the centuries in the official learning centers of Europe until nearly the twentieth century. After the codification of the Twelve Tables the national laws were added to the chant, which was taken up by the Roman schools. No loophole for individual expression here!

In the planning of education for the young the Romans showed a different purpose than that of the Greeks. "They looked not for harmony, proportion, or grace, but for stern utility."[34] According to Graves, girls may have attended the same elementary schools as the boys. One would see here the dawn of co-education, as shown by the following quotation from Martial:

What right have you to disturb me, abominable school-master, object abhorred *by girls and boys alike*? [Italics mine]. Before the crested cocks have broken silence, you begin to roar out your savage scoldings and blows.

(Martial, Book IX, lxviii)

There is no further evidence given than this quotation. However, the fact that the boy is specifically mentioned with the girl would seem to support this assumption.

Of this we can be certain: the school was not softer than the home and the relentless tyranny of the father was re-duplicated in the teacher. We learn that severe physical punishment was applied. "The rod . . . , the lash . . . , and the more brutal whip . . . are mentioned as if in fre-quent use in the Roman schoolroom."[35] A variety of highly revealing terms apply to the schoolmasters of Roman time, such as "ferocious," "irascible," "harsh," "bawling," "fond of blows." The degree and nature of the teacher's sadistic be-havior towards his pupils is recorded for all times in a fresco of Herculaneum. It depicts a teacher securing the efficient co-operation of two of his pupils in the beating of a third pupil on his bare back. This is codified and custom-approved sadism, not the impulsive aggression that might come from an exasperated teacher. What with unduly long hours and rigid demands, in addition to the brutality just recounted, school life could not have been a very rewarding experience.

As education progressed from elementary to grammar school, an artistic climate was introduced by way of paint-ings and sculptures displayed about. The curriculum was still exacting, and punishment apparently lost none of its severity.

It seems that discipline softened somewhat during the reign of Augustus (63 B.C.-A.D. 14), and punishment as an exclusive approach to training seems to have been slightly on the wane. Quintilian (A.D. 35-A.D. 95) rose against cor-poral punishment with three main objections: 1. that cor-poral punishment is humiliating and should be reserved for slaves; 2. that if a boy is impervious to verbal remonstrance, physical punishment can only reinforce his deviant behavior; and 3. that with adequate support from his teacher he would not have needed to be punished in the first place. This positive approach to normal behavior and deviant behavior is a landmark in a slowly moving story: the sympathetic understanding of the child's needs.

The Hellenization of Rome subsequent to the conquest of Greece broadened the cultural patterns of Roman society and its educational programs. It also brought on other changes.

We are told that during the Roman Empire (27 B.C.-A.D. 284) family life underwent a profound modification. The mother's influence became almost nil, owing to the handing over of children to nurses and servants. Quintilian's writings are replete with expressions of indignation over the moral corruption of the child. This "moral corruption" he interprets as growing from overindulgence and the witnessing by children of the license and amorality of their parents.

The unfortunate children learn these vices before they know that they are vices; and hence, rendered effeminate and luxurious, they do not imbibe immorality from schools, but carry it themselves into schools.[36]

During the period described by Gibbon in *The Decline and Fall of the Roman Empire,* from the third century A.D., there was a rapid deterioration of Roman family and society, and infanticide is known to have increased to inordinate proportions.

We cannot overemphasize the influence on the societies that were to follow of the Roman family pattern and its interrelations with the Roman Law. The absolute right of the father to give and take life; to control, coerce, and punish on his own responsibility and judgment; his readiness to utilize, exploit, and transact on the person of his child—all these are strangely reminiscent of customs existing during the Middle Ages and on through the nineteenth century. Do we not find the child sometimes consigned to a short destiny because his father or some odd member of the social group had so decided? Do we not find the child at the end of the nineteenth century in such a plight that laws had to be passed to protect him from slave labor in mines, glass-blowing, and other industrial works?

Roman Law, owing to Rome's successive invasions and

conquests, permeated the laws and customs of European countries. Events of great significance from the point of view of the child's status in society are found, for instance, in the history of England, France, and Germany from medieval times up to the twentieth century. These events reflect conditions analogous to the subjection the Roman child experienced in his times. The Victorian father has been painted as an ogre. Modern commentators are prone to present him as a despotic, unchallenged figure in his family. Seen in the light of his predecessors, the Victorian father—walrus moustache, top hat, cane, and all—seems quite benign, even if the cane was impulsively brandished in moments of anger. Indeed, by contrast he appears warm and highly concerned about his children and their welfare.

The tale of cruelty and indifference toward the child continues and becomes intensified in the barbarian periods which preceded the Middle Ages in most of Europe. In these times killings and massacres involved society as a whole. It would be difficult to single out historical facts pertaining specifically to the fate of children, although contemporaneous tales are not reticent on the subject.

THE MIDDLE AGES (476-1500)

The Middle Ages were times of superstition and religiosity. The clergy played an important role as educators, physicians, and, in general, as leaders of opinion. It is fitting, therefore, that we look into the writings and teachings of St. Augustine (A.D. 356-430).[87] These had a strong influence on the monks and nuns to whom so many children were entrusted, and one would like to learn that the children reaped some benefit from them.

The concept of original sin is elaborated upon. In his eyes the infant was "selfish," even in the desire to suckle. He was innocent only because physically unable to harm. Augustine is aware of sibling rivalry, giving, for instance, a vivid description of hatred in the eyes of an older child witnessing the younger sibling at his nurse's breast. He sees these phenomena as universal. In his estimation "guilt and responsibility" fall, not on the mothers or nurses, but on the child. He would expect a young child to be able to reason out the futility of his jealousy on the basis of the "abundance of the supply." He sees the child as guilty of the "hateful feelings," but he is ready to forgive him because of their evanescent quality.

> Even though it be a vice and a considerable vice, one will suffer it in children and love them nonetheless because one knows that it will be outgrown with time. (My transl.)

Here the child appears not in the abstract or for didactic discussions, but as a concrete human being equipped with feelings. Although Augustine's observations need reinterpretation, we know that he is fully aware of the child's feelings, their subtle nuances, and their sometimes dramatic intensity.

We read of the young child making every effort to learn in order to avoid whipping. Recalling his own childhood, Augustine shows an amazing insight into his feelings and the motivation behind the behavior of adults. After stating that he was intelligent and possessed of a good memory, he adds,

> but I liked to play and amuse myself, and my teachers were punishing me, although they did the same on their own, since what grown men call business affairs are really only amusements. Thus the teachers, as childish as the children themselves, punish them for what they have in common with children, and nobody sympathizes with either the ones or the others of these children. (My transl.)

Exposed as a child to activities and diversions at an adult level, he later reproaches himself for having yielded to accepted and encouraged customs which he now sees as reprehensible. He elaborates on the child's not being as innocent as he is thought to be, and revels in the recounting of "sinful" thoughts and actions which, as he felt, were a reflection of a corrupted adult world. The complexity of a child's inner life is here vividly revealed and analyzed with a sharp-edged scalpel, but with guilt feelings which blunt the total effect.

He is intensely preoccupied with "original sin" and the strong desire to redeem himself. We see the man of the Middle Ages similarly preoccupied with original sin. Superstitions, religious rites, and obsessive thoughts spring from this same preoccupation with self-punishment and salvation.

From historical accounts of the Middle Ages it is clear that a child's life was not worth much. The violent and primitive impulses of the father's behavior toward his children is illustrated in a tale recorded by Sir Samuel Dill.[38] Following the stealing of a horse by some stranger, a man became outraged and his wife attempted to pacify him. "Their son, who seconded his mother's prayer, narrowly escaped death from his father's battle-axe."

We read of the plagues which ravaged the populations and of a "smallpox" type of disease which was particularly devastating to children. Their desire to live may not have been at the optimum, and their physical resistance was undoubtedly at a low ebb. We see large crowds of people turning for miraculous cures for an extraordinary variety of diseases and symptoms to one church or another. The miraculous cures were, after all, not so miraculous or numerous, since we also hear of the rapid spreading of epidemics followed by death, of the insufficient supply of coffins, and of corpses burned in mass in trenches. Intense faith, visions, and all kinds of hallucinatory experiences among children are as evident as among adults, and perhaps more so.

Children are used as pawns, and we read, for instance, of the victor receiving the orphaned daughter of the vanquished as his share of the booty. Only eight years of age and beautiful enough to attract the attention of the victor, her fate was sealed on short notice.

According to some historians it would appear that the family in the Middle Ages took on solidity and developed into a unit, "perhaps the simplest and most individual form which up to that time history had known."[39] This point wants reexamination in the light of customs later to be discussed: the common phenomenon of "oblat disposition" of the children and the general practice of placing children from all levels of society outside of their homes.

Of the oblat more will be said. At this point let it be recalled that, although it did not mean physical destruction as did exposure, the selection for oblats was a form of exclusion of the child from family life and the obliteration of all his chances for ever being a part of it.

The prevalence of *nourrices* and nurses directly reflects a lack of wholeness in the family unit. Nowadays, when a child is in need of a mother substitute, and adoption is not considered, the foster mother steps in. The term itself implies that the temporary parental figure is expected to be a mother. The word *nourrice* applied both to women now called wet nurses and to foster mothers. However, the mercenary quality of the *nourrices* is transparent in historical accounts: if they were not paid they were just as likely to let the children die. Apart from extremely rare instances, it is doubtful that this could happen today. *Nourrices* in the Middle Ages represented a vast body with influence and prerogatives. They were also exploited, and we find that later it was necessary to codify their duties and privileges.

A statement about the "absolute equality" of the family is also questionable.[40] The general opinion is that the father was still omnipotent, that his elder son was called upon to succeed him and was, therefore, next in importance, and that in the lower classes livestock took precedence over wives and children.

> Many consider not the value of a boy or a girl, and many folk who have them hold them of little worth, and when their wife brings forth a little girl, they cannot suffer her, so small is their discretion! Why, there are men who have more patience with a hen, which layeth a fresh egg daily, than with their own wedded wife.[41]

Numerous are the accounts of the superstitions relating to children and of the involved incantations and rites performed to free them of possession. Hallucinatory experiences in children are commonly reported. To be sure, not in such terms, but as miraculous visions, experiences with the devil, and a variety of mystico-religious experiences.

In tracing mental illness and its treatment through the ages, Zilboorg and Henry have described the vast increase of mental illnesses in epidemic form at the end of the fourteenth and beginning of the fifteenth century which compelled the state to take sweeping measures against them.

> The number of mentally sick individuals, as well as the severity of psychopathological epidemics, became so imposing that toward the close of the fourteenth century and at the beginning of the fifteenth century the State not only had to take swift and drastic cognizance of the danger, but it had to formulate its stand toward these frightful happenings. . . . By the middle of the fifteenth century . . . in this religious atmosphere of anxious intensity and combative religious fervor medical psychology became a part of codified demonology, and the treatment of the men-

tally ill became for the most part a problem of legal procedure. The darkest ages of psychiatry set in.[42]

The fervor of purification involved all ages and both sexes. We see that boys and girls between the ages of nine and eleven were convicted and destroyed by flame.

Children of the privileged classes received a well-rounded education, both boys and girls being, like the Roman child, trained at home until seven or eight by their mother. At this time the boy was turned over to the lord of some castle or to some high churchman. As a page he was distinguished from the "inferior members of the household" only in that he was taught by the lady and the lord.

Girls were also brought to some castle where they too received an education. Some of them, indeed, became as proficient in Latin verse writing as were the boys. According to one authority,[43] the girl in Medieval times often applied herself to "bookish learning," and during the eleventh and twelfth centuries co-education "was not unknown."

Apart from individual differences in native abilities and within the limitations of social status, the modern child enjoys a large measure of self-determination about his own future. To the Medieval child this would have been totally unintelligible. The latter had nothing to say of his state. His future was mapped out by his father at the child's birth or in the few years following. But even the father did not act exclusively on his own volition; he responded to the pressure of religious and social forces which were overwhelming.

No matter whose responsibility it was, children were frequently offered as oblats in monasteries and convents. The usual age was seven, but sometimes four or five. The oblation was absolutely binding, since renouncing monastic life would mean excommunication, "with all temporal and spiritual penalties attached."[44] Excommunication then was a living death. The education of oblats was, if anything, more rigorous, and physical punishment more severe, than anything ever found in Sparta. With a radically different motivation, the results were the same.

For Children everywhere need custody with discipline and discipline with custody. And be it known that this is all their discipline, either to be beaten with rods, or that their hair should be stoutly plucked; never are they disciplined with kicks, or fists, or the open hand, or in any other way.[45]

Severity of treatment applied as well to the boys attending the monastery for the exclusive purpose of education without oblat vows.

The concept of original sin, for which dire punishment must be suffered, is still in force; but the understanding and sympathetic words of Augustine have been forgotten.

So far as self-determination goes, the girl's lot was no more enviable. We are told that even the king's daughter did not escape the implacable oblat destiny. In addition, while marriages were arranged for children at all social levels, it was of particular social importance in the hierarchies. Among others, we find Charles the Bold married at the age of six.

If we now go into the question of medical care of the child, rather frightful pictures come before our eyes. Here documentation proves very difficult, since, as pointed out by Dorothy Louise Mackay,

> People of the Middle Ages preferred small houses to large hospitals. They sought to reconstruct the family home. That is why a great many of them escape historical research. (My transl.)[46]

A hospital then was a sort of waste-basket where the sick, the old, the young and very young, the blind, the leprous, passing pilgrims, and unfortunates of all kinds were thrown together, five or six to a bed. There were no hospitals specifically for sick children, not even special wards. When a woman came to the hospital for her own care, her young progeny came along to be distributed among places which happened to be available in the beds. Children who had been abandoned or were admitted because of illness were completely assimilated to the adults, bedded with them, and given the same treatment.

There were innumerable children abandoned as newborns or at a very young age. The Church soon rose in alarm and made it possible for the infants to be saved. The doors of churches and convents became common usage as places of abandonment. The number of children left at monasteries and convents is not known, but a note found in Bonzon[47] indicates that five to six thousand children, mostly born in Paris, were brought yearly to the house founded later by Vincent de Paul (1577-1660).

In the Middle Ages, abandoned children became serfs. And we shall see that this compulsory measure was abolished only at the end of the eighteenth century.

The historical and religious significance of the adults' crusades is well known. The children's counterpart, its overtones of meaning, and its social ramifications need emphasis. Its development follows a pattern which is familiar through the Middle Ages: hallucinatory experience of one member who becomes leader, mass reaction set off in a highly suggestible medium of followers, crescendo of passionate activities, and dissolution of the group with untold damage to the individual.

In the early summer of the year 1212, a young shepherd boy in France told other shepherd boys that in a recent vision he had seen the Lord, who sat down, shared bread with him, and told him that the cross might be redeemed only by innocent children.[48, 49] Now, many young children in those times had visions. Often a child felt compelled to share his visions with someone in his environment, which proved to be safe or not so safe depending on the interpretation at the receiving end. He might be thought to be especially chosen to carry out some consecrated work, or perhaps to be possessed. The latter might set in motion the whole process of purification of his soul.

The shepherd boy, Steven, dared to go to the king, bringing a letter which he asserted had been given to him by Christ in person. When the king told him to go home, the boy eloquently pleaded his desire to imitate Peter the Hermit, who had led the first adult crusade. A movement was then initiated which could have taken place only in Medieval times. Religious fervor alone cannot explain it, and the complexity of the factors involved can hardly be reconstructed.

The boy proceeded toward the south of France. Without benefit of the means of mass communication that are available today, the expedition gained momentum, the grapevine and the witnessed movement being sufficient stimuli. A famished, poorly clothed, disparate crowd of thirty thousand children under twelve years of age reached the Mediterranean coast.

There were simple peasants, whose parents had willingly let them go, also boys of noble birth who had slipped away from home, also girls, young priests, and a few older pilgrims.[50]

What sort of relationship did these children have with their parents, that, religious purpose or no, could allow them to start on such a strange voyage? True, the parents themselves were fanatically religious and may have been prejudiced by the missionary character of the movement. Nevertheless, it speaks for loose parent-child relationships that a large number of young children could start on such an unrealistic adventure, facing certain doom, without the parent's willingness or ability to interfere.

A large number of them, offered an opportunity to sail across the Mediterranean, saw in this gratuitous offer a miracle. Seven large boats were used in the process, two of which "with rotten bottoms and torn sails were caught in a storm and wrecked."[51] The children who survived were landed amidst Moslems, who tortured them. The latter fact was learned through the return, some eighteen years later, of a survivor.

A similar phenomenon took place in Germany very shortly thereafter. They were seven thousand when they reached Italy, having also followed a boy leader, Nicholas. At the start they had been succored by their own people, but when they returned, having failed in their mission, the attitude of the people toward them had changed.

Nicholas's followers perished of hunger and thirst, and froze in the forest when they were not attacked by wild animals. The few who reached their homes were treated ignominiously by the villagers. The maidens that came back to sit at their parents' hearths were mocked and scorned by the maidens who had remained at home. "You have gone forth virgins and returned as harlots."[52]

If as an individual the man of the Middle Ages counted little, the child counted even less. It was not until the end of the eighteenth century that laws were instituted for the prevention of crimes against the child. In particular these laws aimed at stemming the destruction of the newborn, which apparently was practiced on a large scale—easy as it was with no compulsory registration and the utter contempt for the child.

In France an attempt was made (Edict of 1556) to institute very severe penalties for infanticide involving the newborn. The very severity speaks for generalized abuse. This edict, however, was to have little effect, and infanticide progressively increased, reaching its peak at the end of the eighteenth century. Pregnant women had neither legal protection nor medico-social support until approximately the same period, a fact relating not only to the position of women in society, but also to the significance of the child in family and society.

Although he was asked to perform tasks of physical endurance beyond his years, the child was helpless, and during the Middle Ages benevolence was not wasted on the helpless. Zilboorg and Henry have commented on the attitude of Medieval Europe toward the helpless.

The early attitude toward the sick and feeble is suggested by a Prussian law still existent in 1230 which included the following statement: "Be a man laden with sick women, children, brothers, sisters or domestics, or be he sick himself, then let them be where they lie, and we praise him too if he would burn himself or the feeble person."[53]

Historians are in disagreement over the frequency of child sacrifice during the Middle Ages. Yet it is generally agreed that the child was used as a sacrificial offering. Margaret Murray, while acknowledging that many of the pagan rites lingered among the people of Great Britain, even after the Christian Church had been established, states that child sacrifice was rare—actually not reported in England, and only once in Scotland.[54] This is in apparent contradiction with a statement found in another study of hers.[55] In Scotland "it was firmly believed that sacrifices of children took place in all classes of society." The first-born was usually immediately offered to the devil "at a foot of a staircase." Moreover, she alludes to the use as seers of boys under puberty.[56] Questioned by a magician-priest, he was to read answers in a hollowed object, which he was probably hypnotized to fix at length. In the course of presenting witchery symbolism the author gives full details of witchcraft practices and the use of the child for these practices.[57]

Superstition and cruelty, which were very general, did not spare the child. Sir Patrick Hastings tells of a family where two young children were seized with convulsions and stomach pains and were known to have "vomited bent pins and two-penny nails."[58] The suggested remedy was to read the Bible to the children, but whenever the father came to a reference to the Almighty, the convulsions became worse. The whole process was blamed on a village woman who was thought to have exorcised the children.

Elsewhere, a mission preacher, Etienne de Bourbon (1195-1265), spoke of a child of noble family who was offered in sacrifice.[59] The most gruesome details of this sacrifice are given, the mother being depicted as offering her living child to the thrust of purifying needles. The child, thought to be bewitched, was to be sacrificed so that the mother's "own child" could be returned to her. In what form he would be returned is all too clear from the fatal outcome. The preacher adds,

after which these murderous mothers would take the child and lay him naked at the foot of the tree upon the straw of his cradle; and taking two candles an inch long they lighted them at both ends from a fire and thus the white hot candles would oftentimes burn the children alive.

Numerous records indicate that witches engaged in a form of cannibalism, which is variously described. Some writers insist that the children used for the witches' broth were usually already dead. It was believed that by eating the flesh of an unbaptized baby "who had never spoken articulate words" the witch would be able to keep quiet under torture.

In order not to confess . . . they make on the Sabbath a paste of black millet with the powder made from the dried liver of an unbaptized child; it has the virtue of taciturnity; so that whoever eats it will never confess.[60]

The question of whether the child was alive or dead when used for such purposes is left unanswered. But there is more than a hint in contemporary documents. Zilboorg and Henry, for instance, refer to the records of a witches' trial which took place in Switzerland during the fifteenth century. Some witches were accused of having devoured thirteen infants. The interrogation of one of the witches is quoted at length; a passage about the manner of securing the infants would leave grave doubts that the children were dead when seized.

"This is the manner of it. We set our snare chiefly for un-baptized children, and even for those that have been baptized, especially when they have not been protected by the sign of the Cross and prayers . . . and sleeping by their parents' side, in such a way that they afterwards are thought to have been overlain or to have died some other natural death."[61]

Witches nowadays are mild figures associated in our minds with Hallowe'en and other merrymakings. Let us not forget that they were very real and powerful for the Middle Ages man. This is seen in the descriptions of the sinister refinements used by the witches in their preparations. Again, when interrogated at the witches' trial, the witch gave this candid account:

"Then we secretly take them from their graves, and cook them in a cauldron until the whole flesh comes away from the bones to make a soup which may easily be drunk. Of the more solid we make an unguent which is of virtue to help us in our arts and pleasures and our transportation; and with the liquid we fill a flask or skin, whoever drinks from which, with the addition of a few other ceremonies, immediately acquires much knowledge and becomes a leader in our sect."[62]

According to all authorities, devils and witches were a very general plague in Germany, Switzerland, and France. When they were finally tracked down at the end of the fifteenth century, it was by the tens of thousands that they were burned, hanged, and destroyed in one way or another. The proliferation of witches and devils, not always in so concrete a form, is nothing short of amazing. To quote Zilboorg and Henry,

St. Fortunatus labored over a possessed man until he cast the very last devil out of him, bringing the total for one unfortunate person to 6,670.[63]

It is granted that children of any century cannot escape the prejudice and customs of their times and their families, and to a degree accept them as a matter of fact, but the child in the Middle Ages was getting more than his share by the very virtue of his weakness and helplessness. We have seen him a common victim of witchcraft, we have seen that nothing protected him from destruction at birth, and we also know that abandonment was so frequent that measures had to be instituted by the Church to save children from physical destruction.[64] Not that saving them meant the promise of a full and happy life, since abandoned children were in some countries doomed to a state of serfdom,[65] in others to a no-better fate.

Modern psychology has brought out the enormous importance of "mothering" of the infant, and the grave consequences attending the loss of the mother (or an adequate mother substitute). Ribble and Spitz, whose work will be discussed later, have been instrumental in establishing this basic foundation of normal development of the child.[66, 67]

Let us pause at this time and ask—in one whose life was prized so little, who was so often handed out indiscriminately to others than his mother, who was in a constant state of anxiety and fear of damnation, who was threatened with punishment for sinful thoughts he was assumed to have—in such a one, could there be a strong urge to live? True, Heaven was promised him, if he duly repented and redeemed his soul, but in the meantime he must live.

We are familiar with the high mortality of children during past ages, particularly during medieval times, although we are not acquainted with exact figures, since there is no reliable check on the total population or the number of births. In

62

Montaigne (1533-1592) we find descriptions of conditions which, characteristic though they be of the Middle Ages, had persisted through the sixteenth century.[68] He refers in particular to the ravages of death through one child population. Of his own eight children, only one lived on, at least past the age of six.

Mention of the survival of one out of five, or a few out of ten or fifteen or more children in a family is not uncommon in chronicles of the times. We are told that physical agents, epidemics, infections due to the lack of hygienic conditions, and malnutrition were responsible for infant mortality. Referring again to the works of modern psychologists and the emphasis they have placed on the need for mothering, the explanation generally given for the high mortality seems inadequate. Let us not overlook the devastating effect of the indifference and even the cruelty which were shown the child during the Dark Ages.

THE RENAISSANCE

The Renaissance spreads over three centuries, the fourteenth through the sixteenth, with a staggering that places Italy first, then in turn France and England—the three countries which have been arbitrarily selected for our survey of child life throughout this period.

Italy. The status of women rose in several aspects. The parity of intellectual education of men and women, while it allowed exchanges on an equal basis, did not mean a greater emotional closeness. There was a reinforcement and unification of the patriarchal family of early Roman society. The father still had authority, but did not dictate his will as he had earlier.

> Nothing is considered of so much importance as education, which the head of the house gives not only to the children, but to the whole household. He first develops his wife from a shy girl, brought up in careful seclusion, to the true woman of the house, capable of commanding and guiding the servants.[69]

Through such means were achieved a closeness and a unity within the family which had been unknown until then. Burkhardt points to the dislocation of the home during the

Middle Ages, contrasting it sharply with the unification which was later achieved. "The spirit of the Renaissance first brought order into domestic life."[70]

It is clear from contemporary accounts that the mother was recognized for the first time as a very important foundation of the home and a force in the character-building of children. A chronicle of the fifteenth century, one of many, quoted by Maud F. Jerrold, contains detailed descriptions of the duties of the family members toward one another:

> The home is the great educational force, and the well-being of the home is dependent on the character and ability of its head: the husband is to be the head but the wife has a very distinct and honourable position.[71]

A modern touch is seen in a custom reported by this historian. The mother was very close to the child during his early years, while the father was more remote. But he soon was called upon to take a greater share of the moral upbringing. This transfer was both advocated and generally in use.

Education was of great concern in Italian society of this period. We see evidence of this in the multiplicity of treatises on education which appear toward the end of the fifteenth century. Education was not only broader, but efforts were made to render it attractive to the child. It was suggested that toys and pictures and bright colors be made part of the teaching process of young children.[72] Thus, subjects were brought to the child's level of perception through the senses—a far cry from the picture of school in ancient Rome. Corporal punishment was condemned on the ground that a child should be handled with love, not through fear.

Several educators whose reputation has come down to our age devised and carried out very modern methods. Their sphere of activity was limited, but not restricted to the privileged classes. One of them, Vittore dai Ramboldoni (1397-1446), tutor at a court in northern Italy, organized a school where not only children of noble birth were taught, but also gifted children of poor origin. He was fully aware of individual differences in native abilities and the need to adjust his teaching to them.[73]

He had a great eye for the aptitude and bent of each pupil and when he discerned any special gift, he would adjust time and method accordingly; nor would he press learning upon the unwilling scholar: having once given him a fair trial, he would say that all had not the same capacity for study and that some other gift must be looked for.[74]

The atmosphere of the school was cheered by frescoes of children at play. The sensory approach anticipating Montessori methods was used, as well as specially devised games with a view to making learning easier and more pleasurable. This was for the younger children, but the age range of the pupils was quite wide.

While education was liberal and extensive, the educator never lost sight of the need of the child to relax and enjoy himself. Apart from a formal program, the teacher brought in a personal note by introducing small groups to outdoor life, such as fishing. Rigorous training was in favor but had become part of a well-rounded individual development rather than an all-inclusive requirement. The simple regimen of the pupils was in great contrast to the license and luxury of the adult life around them.

How general this brilliant picture could have been during the Italian Renaissance is difficult to establish. To begin with, the picture applies primarily to northern Italy, and in particular to the upper classes. There is another side to this picture.

It is known that there was still a great deal of superstition, and witches continued to be feared and exorcised. What applied to the end of the Middle Ages also applies here. Barbarian customs, which seem to come straight down from the Roman sacrificial rites and medieval witchcraft, are reflected in the reported story of three shepherd boys of the district of Aquapendente.[75] Curious to determine just how a man was hanged, they raised one of their companions on their shoulders, placing his head in a noose. A wolf interrupted their "experiment." The two boys ran, leaving their companion hanging from the tree. When they returned, they found him dead and buried him. The dead boy's father learned of the tragic outcome. He killed the culprit with a knife, cut out his liver, and entertained the boy's father with it.

Dual characteristics of culture and barbarism we find also during the English and French Renaissance.

England. We are given to understand that education of children, not only at the level of the privileged classes, but also among the poor, was not neglected during the English Renaissance.[76] Public schools, in the English sense of the word, had preceded the creation of the Dame schools. The extent of the student population is not known, but on the assertion of one historian,[77] "Half the population was illiterate." Girls did not fare as well as boys. "What little education they had was given them by their brothers' tutors, in the case of the well-to-do, but most poor girls had no education at all," whereas boys were put to learn very early. The atmosphere of the home was not conducive to warm relations between parents and child. Parents were distant and expected strict obedience.

Like his Medieval counterpart, the child of the Renaissance was expected to perform tasks beyond his physical strength and emotional maturity. Poor children received a smattering of knowledge and were early apprenticed to various trades.

Superstition was still rampant. It was the custom for women to wear charms before their baby's birth. And midwives were required to swear that they would not change the newborn by sorcery. Murray points out that the most brilliant minds of the sixteenth century believed in the evidence brought out at the witches' trials,[78] and chronicles of the time contain many stories of bewitching and exorcising.

Child sacrifice is said to have been still in existence, and Murray quotes Reginald Scot (1584) on child sacrifice:

"If there be anie children unbaptized, or not guarded with the signe of the crosse, or orizons; then the witches may or doo catch them from their mothers sides in the night, or out of their cradles, or otherwise kill them for their ceremonies."[79]

He must have been convinced of the prevalence of these practices, since he writes,

"This must be an infallible rule, that euerie fortnight, or at the least euerie moneth, each witch must kill one child at the least for hir part."[80]

The lanes of towns in that period were not safe, and hordes of boys who appear as various degrees of what we would today call juvenile delinquents roamed the streets. This situation was to worsen seriously during the seventeenth and eighteenth centuries.

France. The Renaissance in France again presents the dual pattern of brilliance in literary and artistic achievements on the one hand, and the continuance of barbarian customs on the other. In our search for the emotional climate generated during this period for the child, we must not lose sight of the fact that witchcraft and superstition continued unabated through the seventeenth and even the eighteenth century.

Education continued in monasteries and nunneries much on the same patterns we have noted for the Middle Ages. We can assume that the conditions of family life have not improved. Let us turn, for instance, to Montaigne. Here we are not so much concerned about his philosophy of education, which marked a definite step forward, but about his observations on the mores of the time and his experience in his own family life. Take, for instance, his observation regarding the high infantile mortality, already referred to. He laments that all his children but one died at the *nourrice* home, but also expresses his helplessness before the universally accepted custom of placing children with the *nourrice. "Ils me meurrent tous en nourrisse."* He rises against physical violence toward children which is general, the very young included, and insists that a child can be raised without it.

I have not seen other effect of whipping than to weaken and cower the soul or make it more maliciously stubborn and antagonistic. Do we want to be loved by our children? Do we wish to prevent them from wishing our death? . . . Then let us mould that life reasonably, at least for what is in our power. For that we would not marry so young that our age come almost to be equal to theirs. (My transl.)[81]

Montaigne saw the meaning of the early years in the building of the personality. The importance of habit-formation during the early years of life is emphasized, with the bitter additional comment that, unfortunately, these years by custom are under the influence of nurses. He gives very dramatic descriptions of children wrenched from their mothers and handed to a *nourrice*, who was often physically and morally unfit. He rises in indignation against this custom which deprives the child of a close relationship with his parents, forcing him to accept a poor substitute, "spurious affection," from his nurses.

His opinion of the capacity and qualification of contemporary parents and educators is not very high, since elsewhere he suggests that children be not left in the hands of their parents, "so foolish and mean can they be." He would select qualified parent-substitutes in the form of tutors. Judging from his account, parents must have been harsh and distant. He begs that children be allowed to call their father not Sir, but Father. The achieving of a softer and more tender relation between parents and children is hoped for.

Hardening the child to physical agents is seen as a necessity, but this should be accomplished without physical violence. Referring to what would be interpreted today as a variety of phobias in children and adolescents, he contrasts the anxiety characteristics of these manifestations with fears that have a definite object. To him the solution would be simple. "Any strange and peculiar manifestation to accepted behavior is avoidable," with early molding at the first opportunity while the personality is still "supple."

Affection from the parents would be one of the best levers in securing compliance as well as returned affection. Probably because of the lack of emotional closeness between parents and children, we find that parents tend to see in their children a source of amusement and diversion. Montaigne comments bitterly on it, and a number of contemporary chronicles echo his opinion. Children are compared to dolls, are called upon to perform on short notice before company, a pernicious habit which may have existed prior to this period, though not apparent through sources consulted. But it is certain that it was to last for several centuries to come, and we find similar comments in historical documents of the eighteenth and nineteenth centuries. During the sixteenth century the performance was on the harpsichord, during the nineteenth it was a piano piece; but in both instances the child was used in the same role of entertainer.

Other bitter comments made by Montaigne on the child's unfortunate place in the family reflect an attitude toward the child which is both novel and heartening. In his thinking about the education of children there is evident an effort at raising the worth and dignity of the child as an individual.

Even for the young child (from pre-school age on) he holds living experience as a teaching approach superior to that of reading and writing. He sees the child capable of reasoning, if he were only encouraged in that direction, rather than having to endure the forced and mechanical infliction of knowledge.

Education of the child, as seen by Montaigne, is better achieved through a gentle approach than through the blind severity which had been in effect for so long. Again, he stands out from his century in his contention that children should not be pushed away from their parents. The cares and preoccupations with matters that concern the home should be shared with the children. In this connection he brings up the story of several adolescent boys who took to robbery, and explains their delinquencies through the father's personality. He was harsh, ungiving, and distant. There is a sort of mellowing of the relationship between parents and children, and much is made of the need for affection both ways, and how it can be nurtured.

While all of this concurred to give a new note in the attitude of the adult toward the child, we are aware that the effect on contemporary mores, and in particular the official education of children, was negligible. We are also aware that this new benevolence and understanding did not protect the child from the atmosphere of demonology, witchcraft, and superstition which was characteristic of this time as well as the Middle Ages. Let us not forget that the practice of child sacrifice by witches is reported during this century also.

Children often became witches—girls more frequently than boys. They are referred to in contemporary writing as child-witches or witch-girls. Demoniacal possession was dealt with in the various manners already described.

It will be recalled that, in glancing over the history of mental illness and its treatment, the statement was made that, prior to the twentieth century, children were not mentioned, except for accounts of rare instances. The following accounts represent the sixteenth-century emergence of children in Zilboorg and Henry's historical survey.[82]

The first child to enter his survey is a young girl, age not given. A black man appeared before her while she was praying at the tomb of her father. In her own words he was Satan. He had attempted to rape her, she had struggled, and he had demanded that she destroy herself. An estimate of the current times places this case as one of possession by an evil spirit. As is pointed out, while a girl in the Middle Ages would tell of and dramatize raping by the devil, her counterpart today would also refer to the black man, but call him a Negro. Ideas of persecution and the drive to self-punishment, including suicide, are similarly found in subjects of both periods. These symptoms were described sometime later as hysterical. They are today considered a part of schizophrenic illness. The visions and voices accompanying them would be part of the hallucinatory experience of the schizophrenic. What is of interest to us, however, is that, as one could have assumed, children suffered mental illness then as they do today.

Zilboorg and Henry quote a case of Weyer, "the man who made the greatest contribution to psychology during the Renaissance." A ten-year-old girl presented symptoms of an alarming nature. She was mute and refused all food, following a period of complete stupor. Malingering, which she achieved with the help of her sister, was revealed through the perspicacity and scientific method of Weyer.

There is also a reference to "a melancholic girl," age not given, who confessed that she was possessed by the spirit of Vergil. Conjurers were called in to exorcise her, but to no avail. Later, she was "cured" by the never-failing remedy of the Middle Ages, purging. "Thus, after the girl's body was purged, the minister of the Church was able to use his means more easily to expel the evil spirit. For, with the natural obstacles

71

removed, he could easily undertake the rest of the treatment."[83]

These authors comment further:

> this method of treating the mentally ill—first putting them in the hands of a physician and then turning them over or leaving them to the good graces of a minister of the Church —has survived till our days, as has the old and worn tradition of considering neuroses inseparably within the province of the Church and its alleged psychotherapeutic wisdom.[84]

Weyer struck a hard blow against witchery, although the effect of his interpretation remained only of academic interest for some time, and a subject of violent controversy. He attacked superstitions and witchcraft practices, reviewing the problem through an analysis of Biblical references and Greek mythology and history.

> He leaves no doubt but that one conclusion is warranted: witches are mentally sick people, and the monks who torment and torture the poor creatures are the ones who should be punished.[85]

His ideas were revolutionary, and it is of no surprise to us that the suggestion of dealing with mass contagion by dispersing the possessed was not followed. He saw the possibility of treating these unfortunates, if they could be approached, not as a group, but in a situation propitious to individual treatment.

COLONIAL AMERICA
(Late Seventeenth and Early Eighteenth Centuries)

Lest it should be thought that the attitudes towards children which have been reported through these pages were a monopoly of European countries, we now turn to Colonial America with a view to learning whether the child in the New World was better favored. A well-documented study by Calhoun provides material.[86] It should be known at the outset that, even though we are coming closer to the twentieth century, documents which have come down to us reveal the same lack of sensitivity to the child's emotional life. We are bound to draw this conclusion when we read,

> Colonial childhood is largely hidden in obscurity. Letters and diaries contain little mention of the children save the record of births and deaths and maladies and the like.[87]

Here letters and diaries are available. But what do they reveal? Dates. Not the everyday observations of children at play, or in their tasks, joys, or griefs.

The family stood well as a unit, bolstered by the dangers from the outside which called for a united front. Families were large. Colonial America had given thought to birth control no more than western Europe. And if birth control had been thought of, it probably would have been severely prohibited.

The stern religion that was characteristic of the settlers was in no way less exacting and punitive than the Catholicism of earlier centuries. As we shall see, the child in the Colonial family was reared in fear of damnation and in morbid preoccupation with the salvation of his soul.

From records which have been available to the historian, it is clear that infant mortality was very high, a fact we are familiar with through our rapid survey of previous centuries in Europe. Calhoun states that "in the barrenness and cold of Massachusetts mortality of infants was frightful."[88] Again, physical agents are solely blamed for the high mortality rate among infants, but here contagious diseases and unhygienic conditions are not in question. We will have occasion to reexamine the fact of high infant mortality, when we get glimpses of the emotional climate in which the child of Colonial times was reared. Statistics as such are unavailable, even if it was general practice for the pilgrims to enter the exact day, hour, and minute of the child's birth so that the horoscope could be attentively followed. Specific examples, however, are given about the number of children who survived in some families; they are highly revealing. For instance Cotton Mather had fifteen children of whom two survived. Three children survived of Judge Sewall's fourteen.

Locke's *Thoughts on Education* was a popular book then, and it appears that following his suggestions meant bringing up children under Spartan rules. For instance, to make children tough it was advised that their feet be moistened with cold water or shod with thin soles. When infants were baptized, it was in a fireless church, even if the ice had to be broken in the font; and one pastor was said to have brought his own infants to the brink of death after immersion in freezing water.

Children were reared in an atmosphere of fear of Hell and anxiety which is reminiscent of the Middle Ages. They had to learn Michael Wigglesworth's *Day of Doom*. In this cheery little piece they were given vivid pictures of children who had died in infancy, pleading that, if Adam, the original sinner, had been saved, so should they be. No mercy was offered them, and children from their earliest years were threatened with the coming of Hell, if they gave vent to any natural impulse. Cotton Mather, whose book *Magnalia Christi Ameri-*

cana exerted a great influence during his time, was also the author of a pamphlet destined for children's entertainment, "Some Examples of Children in Whom the Fear of God Was Remarkably Budding Before They Died."

Of Cotton Mather's approach to the moral education of his own child, we learn directly from him:

> I took my little daughter (aged four) into my study and there told my child that I am to dy shortly and she must, when I am dead, remember everything I now said unto her. I sett before her the sinful condition of her nature and charged her to pray in secret places every day. That God for the sake of Jesus Christ would give her a new heart. . . . I gave her to understand that when I am taken from her she must look to meet with more humbling than she does now she has a tender father to provide for her.[89]

He himself must have lived in a state of anxiety, since Calhoun adds the comment that this scene took place thirty years before Mather's death.

Numerous are the illustrations of children who were similarly raised through fear. To modern man it is probably impossible to fathom the depth of gloom in which a child of this period was living. The devil, the bogey man, the policeman are anemic figures to use for comparison. The fear of Hell was very real and a powerful weapon in the hands of parents and educators.

However, of witchcraft and superstition, as we have followed them in Europe, we find only rare examples. The well-known outburst which took place in Salem, Massachusetts, in 1692 is called to mind. The old pattern of accusations of bewitching by some young and irresponsible individuals is familiar to us. In the new milieu an atmosphere was recreated which was heavily laden with medieval prejudice. Unfounded accusations against nineteen women inexorably led them to the gallows, as it would have during the thirteenth century. It can be fairly assumed that children were not spared the lessons which could be drawn then and there. Leave it to the Puritan preacher contemporary with the "Day of Doom" to exploit such an edifying opportunity.

Again, as in the Middle Ages, we find that young children

were expected to perform feats of learning which today are offered at the high school level. We hear of three-year-old children taught at home to read Latin along with the English language and of four- and five-year-olds reading the Bible. About 1649 an attempt at compulsory education appeared in New England (excluding Rhode Island). It was short-lived owing to demands put upon youth to help in the struggle for survival.

Boys were men at sixteen, served in the militia, and even paid taxes. It is revealing that Governor Winthrop made his fourteen-year-old son executor of his will, being obviously satisfied that he was mature enough to carry the responsibility. Of duties and responsibilities expected from young children, we see ample evidence. Of the privileges, joys, and satisfactions a young child could feed on, we see none. In fact, there was a definite tendency to curb any propensity on the part of the child toward amusement as a dangerous obstacle to his salvation.

We are at least impressed with the fact that parents were highly responsible toward their children and were concerned about them, even if their goal was restricted to the salvation of their soul and was not conducive to the unfolding of their personality. The child's relation to his parents was awe-inspired. He addressed them as "esteemed parent," "honored Sir," and "Madam" and dared not bring out personal requests except in very formal ways such as writing.

Complete obedience and submissiveness on the part of the child were expected. Every facet of his behavior was anticipated and rules were laid down. As appears in a widely circulated book of etiquette, directions about the suitable behavior of children at table read in part as follows:

Never sit down at the table till asked, and after the blessing. Ask for nothing; tarry till it be offered to thee. Speak not. Bite not thy bread but break it. Take salt only with a clean knife. Dip not the meat in the same. Hold not thy knife upright but sloping and lay it down at right hand of plate with blade on plate. Look not earnestly at any other that is eating. When moderately satisfied leave the table. Sing not, hum not, wriggle not. Spit nowhere in the room but in the corner. . . . When any speak to thee, stand up. Say not I have heard it before. Never endeavor to help him out if he tell it not right. Snigger not; never question the truth of it.[90]

Fortunately, underneath the constant needling from parents about behavior there is apparent in Calhoun's account a certain parental warmth and tenderness. The awesome Cotton Mather also wrote a booklet which was much in demand, "A Family Well Ordered, or an Essay to Render Parents and Children Happy in One Another." Needless to say, the scale weighed on the side of the parents even in this kindlier enterprise.

It is a relief to learn of children's mischief at school or in church, even though penalties were dealt out for it. The notebook of a Connecticut justice of that period lists children's offenses under the heading of smiling, laughing (at church), and "enticing others to the same evil."

To the despair of contemporary preachers, extreme puritanism began to wane toward the second half of the seventeenth century; and Reverend Ezekial Rogers wrote in 1657,

Do your children and family grow more godly? I find greatest trouble and grief about the rising generation. Young people are little stirred here; but they strengthen one another in evil by example and by counsel. Much ado have I with my own family.[91]

Colonial laws appeared which aimed to restore the formerly unchallenged parental authority and entrust magistrates with the power to summon offenders and punish them by whipping. "For incorrigible disobedience to parents, the colonists, in accordance with Moses and Calvin, prescribed the death penalty."[92] However, there is no evidence that the penalty was ever carried out.

That the children were an object of close concern to their parents and that the family had tightened up its parent-child relationships by comparison with contemporary western Europe is all too clear. Even though the family milieu was far from ideal for children, the change marks an advance. A

77

tightening up of the family in the face of danger common to all took place in conditions of isolation, which were also binding. Freedom for the child and the right to fulfill his potentialities, however, were to be long in coming.

SEVENTEENTH CENTURY EUROPE

After this brief incursion into Colonial America let us return to the Europe of the seventeenth century. The century division being arbitrary, we can expect that patterns of living will have undergone little change.

France. A reaction to oppressive methods used in monasteries and convents was apparently taking place. Authorities on this period have elaborated upon the breakdown of moral education in children and adolescents during the seventeenth century in France. Aldous Huxley has drawn from an autobiographical account of a seventeenth century youth, who

has left us a document so clinically objective, so completely free from all expression of regret, from any kind of moral judgment, that nineteenth century scholars could publish it only for private circulation and with emphatic comments on the author's unspeakable depravity. For a generation brought up on Havelock Ellis and Krafft-Ebing, on Hirschfeld and Kinsey, Bouchard's book no longer seems outrageous. But though it has ceased to shock, it must still astonish. For how startling it is to find a subject of Louis XIII writing of the less creditable forms of sexual activity in the flat, matter-of-fact style of a modern college girl answering an anthropologist's questionnaire, or a psychiatrist recording a case history.[93]

While this autobiographical record might not be typical of all youths of that period, there is, nevertheless, additional evidence that children were brought up in an atmosphere of sexual promiscuity which was the result of complex factors: the breaking down of authority and discipline of religious educators, the lack of normal outlets for motor and aggressive activities, and the complete absence of privacy in the home—even among the upper classes. The architectural layout of rooms, which were not actually closed rooms, was in part responsible for this state of affairs. The fact is certain that children were under no supervision, as accounts of the period clearly indicate.[94] Even where education would be expected to be at its best, we find, for instance, that the king's eldest son, to become king himself as Louis XIV (1638-1715), was at five years of age entrusted to governesses who paid no attention to him, occupied as they were with their own games of cards or other social activities. Nobody seemed to know or bother to know where he might be, and he was most often found in the company of a little peasant girl. Once he was saved from drowning in one of the fountains only by chance, since nobody was cognizant of his whereabouts. The Duke de Lauzun (1632-1723), one of the nobles closes to the king, has left the following testimony, quoted by Taine.[95]

I was, moreover, like all the children of my age and of my station dressed in the handsomest clothes to go out, and naked and dying with hunger in the house, not through unkindness but through household oversight, disorder, attention being given to things elsewhere.

If one is to judge what the status of the child in the family was among the poorer classes from these glimpses into the aristocracy, then one must acknowledge that the picture was not very bright. Mothers at all social levels are said to have shown little interest in their daughters' education, and it was the custom to have a governess at home or to send the child to a convent. Education continued very sketchy, with convent teachers not adequately qualified. The need for reform in the education of children was urgent, and before the end of the century such reform was to appear with Fénélon and

Mme. de Maintenon. The reform bore mainly on the extension of learning and the softening of punishment.

Some hard-to-kill institutions continued to thrive, such as child marriage and witchcraft, which—in the latter case and according to one authority—included twelve- to sixteen-year-old girls.[97] As we can see, the status of the child in the family and society had not improved.

England. England of the seventeenth century shows no improvement in the child's status. Mitchell gives us a vivid picture of customs and family life during Tudor and Stuart times.[98]

While we get the impression that discipline softened a little for the child under some circumstances, nevertheless compassion and understanding were entirely lacking in the meting out of punishment and the reason for it. John Gwyther, commenting on the social environment at the end of the seventeenth century, writes:

> A country that waved aside the necessity of a police force and protected its citizens by the legal atrocities of the law; courts which unconcernedly sentenced a lad of eight to death for stealing a pot of paint valued at twopence, or deported for life an eleven year old girl who had dressed as a boy and borrowed a neighbor's horse.[99]

It is evident that much depended on the Justice's sympathy whether punishment was mild or severe for antisocial behavior —behavior we would now classify as juvenile delinquency—and referring here to very minor offences, such as stealing eightpence or even less.

In the home, disciplining did not mean the carrying out of the severe corporal punishment we have seen applied consistently. As seen from a passage in Mitchell's *History,* some allowance was made for parental individual differences in the chastising of their children.

> Discipline varied greatly, from the harshness and formalism that compelled little Elizabeth Tanfield only to speak to her mother when kneeling humbly before her, to the tenderness of Endymion Porter who urged his wife to have

81

little George's hair cut short and not to beat him overmuch. Puritans had a firm belief in the rod, and set about whipping the devil out of their children with zeal and fervor, but the urbane George Savile, Marquess of Halifax, gave his daughter quite other advice on bringing up children.[100]

Nevertheless, it cannot be said that, on the whole, the child enjoyed much tenderness from parents or parent substitutes. We have the téstimony of Lady Jane Grey, executed at an age of just over sixteen, "that if she did not do every insignificant action 'even so perfectly as God made the world,' her parents would pinch, slap, and beat her till she thought she was in Hell."[101]

Infant mortality, as on the continent, continued very high during this century in England. Obviously no statistics are available, but, as was the case elsewhere, diaries and letters and old tombstones of the time are revealing in this respect.

Monuments in churches and inscriptions on tombstones show how frequently children died at birth or in the first few years of life; the monument to John Greene in Navestock church records that he had six children "beside some few that died younge," and this could be paralleled in many parts of the country. If this was the case among the upper classes, the children of the poor must have had even less chance of survival, and indeed, the parish registers of the time tell a sad tale.[102]

Efforts at preventing infants' death are evident in the special attention paid to the physical comfort of babies. This applied to the upper classes, and we do not know the extent to which infants were protected from the rigor of unheated houses during the winter.

However cold the rest of the house might be, with the wind sweeping down the long gallery and whistling in the chimneys, the nursery would be snug and warm, and the baby swathed like a chrysalis in his swaddling clothes, lying in his solid wooden cradle stuffed with blankets and feather quilts and pillows, rocked by his nurse's foot before a glowing peat fire, was more likely to be smothered than chilled.[103]

On the authority of Mitchell, "men of the seventeenth century were more natural and affectionate fathers than is sometimes supposed."[104]

Education was given, as formerly, in the public and "petty" schools, the latter to include children of poor families who showed promise. Most children of the poor were automatically excluded, however, since they were occupied at some type of hard physical work to add small wages to the family pittance.

Modern man is confounded by the precociousness of the children of this and previous periods, which enabled some children of three and four to read and express themselves in Latin. Milton (1608-1674) tells of his father's determination to have him pursue the study of humanities. He recalls that at twelve years he almost never went to bed before midnight, having pored since early morning over his texts at the cost of his eyesight and the suffering of headaches.[105] Children did not evince a very keen interest in the forced study they were subjected to, but the achievements attained through this coercion are not less of a wonder to us.

The education of the girl was devised with a very definite object, to prepare her for marriage, which was planned from and sometimes for the childhood years. There is some evidence of co-education in a limited degree, as some schools admitted girls in the lower classes. However, most public schools objected strongly to co-education in the belief that it was "'uncomely and not decent.'"[106]

What about entertainment devised for the children? Relics and mementoes of games and toys for the use of children have been preserved. But let us not forget a choice piece of entertainment of that period, the watching of hangings and tortures. A fourteen-year-old boy, for instance, is cited as having watched a man whipped at a cart-tail and marvelling at his frightful endurance.[107] On the continent, children were also treated with the witnessing of public executions and tortures; only the form varied.

Another questionable form of entertainment was the accepted custom of taking the children to visit the mentally ill at Bedlam and other asylums. Note in passing the tagging along of children within the radius of parental activities. As is well known, the mentally ill were chained, starved, beaten, and kept in filth and darkness. The visit was a routine holiday program akin to a visit to the zoo in our days. The difference is that strict rules apply to the teasing and tormenting of animals, whereas of the period we speak, teasing was not only legitimate but considered more or less a duty, since the insane were thought more or less possessed. Cowper tells us that the Bedlam visit was a favorite occupation for the Westminster boys, and that, although he was not himself "altogether insensible" of their miseries, "the madness of them had such a harmonious air and displayed itself in so many whimsical freaks, that it was impossible not to be entertained."[108]

This attitude toward the mentally ill was general among adults, but the fact that children were included reveals in the parents a lack of awareness of the child's sensitivity to traumatic experiences. However exhilarating the spectacle may have been to the surrounding adults, one can easily assume that a child would project himself into the situation of the victim, with resultant anxiety. With the fear of death and damnation a constant companion, the anxiety could be overwhelming. We do not find in records that anyone did perceive the likely turmoil within the child.

Belief in witchery is long-lived, as we can see from many references to the possessed and the demoniacal. The trial of a child witch in 1661 is mentioned by Murray.[109] While the peak of persecution of witches is considered by Mitchell to have been reached toward the end of the 17th century, the reader will recall that the last executions of witches on the continent took place at the end of the eighteenth century. Obviously, there were sporadic incidents of belief in witches in rural districts in England, since Mitchell describes a Dorset man accusing a neighbor of bewitching his pig in 1926.[110]

While we are given no insight into the emotional life of children of the time, it is all too evident that the emotional climate of that day was still oppressive, inhibiting and, to a degree, cruel. The relation between parents and children was still devoid of warmth, and the child went on living in a world of submission very close to abjectness.

EIGHTEENTH CENTURY

France. The eighteenth century in France is a turning point in the condition of the child as a part of the family and society. Apparent is the marked disparity between the aristocracy and the living conditions of the poorer classes. One of the results of the French Revolution was to level social differences and raise the socio-political status of the lower classes, a result which was not immediate.

From a study of Duval we learn that during the eighteenth century the number of illegitimate births and children's abandonments reached such proportions that severe measures were taken to protect the child.[111] Recommendations made by the general controller of finance, Orry, toward the end of the century are to the effect that Justices must provide for the care of foundlings until the age of seven. When children have reached this age, it is suggested that they be put to work with peasants until twenty years of age. In this legal document a comment is made by Orry which appears cynical to us but it can be traced to the Law of the Twelve Tables on the use and exploiting of a child as part of the patrimony:

A child of seven begins to render some services on a farm land. And when he would reach a more advanced age he would become a servant to whom one would not pay wages and who would be the more useful as he would be held in an entire dependence of his master. (My transl.)[112]

Historians agree on the breaking down of moral values at

this time throughout all classes, but particularly at the top. Whenever abuses are loudly crying, reforms and laws to deal with them are not far behind.

Foundlings in great number were entrusted to *nourrices;* and a code was formulated in 1781 to protect them against the exploitations of agents, who played middle men and extorted high fees from them, and the infants in their care.

There was no absolute safeguard of the child's life until the onset of the French Revolution, when specific laws were formulated for his protection. Indeed, we get some idea of the ruthlessness applying to the handling of these unfortunate children in a vivid description by Bonzon. "The children entrusted to the *nourrices* were piled up in farm wagons and thus taken sometimes to great distances."[113] We are informed that, if parents were lax in the payment of mensualities, the nurses were apt to neglect the children, with the possibility of death as an outcome. The mortality among these children was very high, as the following figures attest. From 1776 to 1790 one hundred thousand children were received in a foundling hospital. Of these only fifteen thousand survived.[114]

When the children reached the age of seven, it was decided whether they would remain for another nine or ten years with the nurses, who received a modest fee for their upkeep. The majority did not stay on, however, and returned to the foundling hospital, from which they were directed to special institutions. They could stay there until the age of twelve, then were hired out as apprentices to various trades, still under the supervision of the institution. It is known that more than three quarters ran away "despite the good lessons in religion which they had received."[115]

It is at this point that we see how the treatment of juvenile delinquency was carried out during the eighteenth century. There were two types of receiving centers for the "incorrigible"—prison, and what would be called today a reform school. The children who rebelled were sent to one or the other, depending on the severity of their misbehavior. In either institution they became part of a desperate crowd of criminals, the insane, epileptics, beggars, and what were known then as incorrigible children.

Taine speaks of a disintegration of the family, particularly in the upper classes.[116] The remoteness between parents and children is revealed by the very forms of language and the outward marks of respectfulness which are characteristic of that period. A number of autobiographical accounts left by members of the aristocratic classes give a uniform picture of children abandoned to servants and virtual strangers to their parents.

If and when parents took notice of them, it was often for the sake of their amusement and their friends' amusement. They were used like dolls and puppets, incongruously dressed for theatrical roles they were to play and perfunctorily dismissed at the end of their performance. They might be called back on short notice to exhibit their talent at music or other skills, all to the amusement and benefit of the assembled company.

Paternal authority was absolute. A father could have his uncomplying and rebellious son locked up for a period of time. As commented by Bonzon,

> The child and his family escaped the jurisdiction of the law; so long as his parents did not make attempts against his life they could give him the education they wanted and hire him out for any kind of work. (My transl.)[117]

Here again we recognize the indelible stamp of the Law of the Twelve Tables.

Abuses are suffered just so long; then, inevitably, reforms are generated to stem their ravages. Thus the work of Rousseau (1712-1778) appeared.[118] Rousseau took nature as a model and attempted to free children from the restrictive influences which had dwarfed and twisted their natural development. He wished to reinstate the mother in the home in a position of dignity and moral importance, not only so far as children were concerned, but as a way of consolidating the marriage unit. "When women are once more true mothers, men will become true fathers and husbands."[119] He must have felt his own inadequacy as a father, since we know that he placed his out-of-wedlock children in a foundling hospital, yet wrote, "He who cannot fulfill the duties of a father has no right to be a father."[120]

A very important and novel conception emerges of the joy derived from the very presence of children, which can help to solidify the father-mother relationship.

> Let mothers only vouchsafe to nourish their children, and our manners will reform themselves. . . . The attractions of home life present the best antidote to bad morals. The bustling life of little children, considered so tiresome, becomes pleasant; it makes the father and the mother more necessary to one another, more dear to one another; it draws closer between them the conjugal tie.[121]

He grows indignant over the patterns of training that were then current which twist the child into an "artificial creature."

At the age of six or seven he was passed on to a tutor who "teaches him everything except to know himself, everything but how to live and how to make himself happy."[122] The thought that the child has a right to happiness, that he be given a chance to enjoy and develop his natural gifts was indeed revolutionary. We find in Rousseau many words of wisdom about the meaning of children (words touching upon many phases of the child's early life) which would appear modern even today. To quote only a few of his observations and exhortations:

> All children are weaned too early. The proper time is indicated by their teething. . . . I do not disapprove of a nurse's amusing the child with song, and with blithe and varied uses. But I do disapprove of her perpetual deafening him with a multitude of useless words, of which he understands only the tone she gives them. . . . Children who are too much urged to speak have not time sufficient for learning either to pronounce carefully or to understand thoroughly what they are made to say.[123]

The new freedom Rousseau would give to the child is tempered with a scrutiny into the dangers of excessive release. Reformers are sometimes given to leap to extremes in combatting abuses which have aroused them. Not so with him.

In the formulation of his concepts he avoids this danger, thus attaining a balance not commonly found in reformers. He has noted the feeling of omnipotence in the child, from which the child must mature by accepting frustrations—in fact, by utilizing them as a means of growth.

> The child who has only to wish in order to obtain his wish thinks himself the owner of the universe. . . . The surest way to make a child unhappy is to accustom him to obtain everything he wants to have. . . . Accustomed to seeing everything give way before them, how surprised they will be on entering the world to find themselves crushed beneath the weight of that universe they have expected to move at their own pleasure.[124]

Releasing the child does not mean complete license. It is a well-regulated freedom. His counsel, "over-strictness and over-indulgence are equally to be avoided,"[125] might have been lifted out of a modern textbook of child psychology.

Throughout, Rousseau refers to "Nature" as his teacher. "Nature intends that children shall be children before they are men. . . . Let the over-strict teacher and the over-indulgent parent both learn the lesson of Nature herself."[126]

His amazing capacity to project himself into the child's mind gave him an awareness of pressures put on the child—pressures which took no account of the young child's intellectual immaturity. Sensory perceptions, images, are a child's riches; not abstract ideas and pedantic knowledge which formal educators have viciously pressed upon him.

It was long after Rousseau's death that his ideas had any influence on practices of education. His writings, however, aroused an immediate interest in the child as an individual, and it came about that children were more fully noticed.

England. In England education retained the standards previously described. Some changes were taking place, but they were not of great importance. The education of girls tended away from domestic skills toward social niceties.[127]

Classical education for the boys had been further intensified, but there is evidence that this was not altogether to the taste of the pupils. Advertisements of the time reflect the frequency of runaways, with penalties threatening the child, and rewards offered to the finder. At twelve years a boy's thoughts turned to the sea, and it is a commentary on the times that he generally could put them into action. A twelve-year-old apparently could hire himself out for work with no questions asked.

The charity schools, which appear to represent an attempt at general, though not compulsory, education, were created during the reign of Queen Anne. But we see the Law of the Twelve Tables and its defining of the use and exploitation of the child lurking behind the curriculum. A writer of the eighteenth century, Mandeville, vents his view on the education of the poor. In an *Essay on Charity Schools,* 1723, he writes:

> Men who are to remain and end their days in a Laborious, Tiresome, and Painful station of Life, the sooner they are put upon it at first, the more patiently they'll submit to it for ever after.[128]

From some reports of the time, the utilitarian purpose of these schools is unmistakable. In one such school thirty little girls were steadily at work on lace from six in the morning till six at night. The exploitation of children in the poorer classes has its parallel with the child's condition on the continent. The child continued to be considered not so much as a human being but as a useful implement for economic and practical necessities.

William Blake (1757-1827) has evoked in his writings images of his childhood, stirring memories which, for all their unique creative quality, must be part of his contemporaries' experience. At the age of seven he began to work in a silk mill, where he was unable to operate the machine without the help of lifts. One day he woke up in terror, thinking that he was late for work because of the unusual brilliance of the atmosphere due to snowing.

> I darted out in agonies, and, from the bottom of Full street to the top of Silkmill lane, not two hundred yards, I fell nine times. Returning, it struck two. As I now went with care, I fell but twice.[129]

His brother, possibly because he was a little more sturdy, put in fourteen hours a day at the same age, and information is given that for this inhuman toil he received the fabulous sum of one shilling a week.

Workhouses, which had been created for a nondescript crowd of vagrants, received women and children as well. The children's schedule covered an eleven-hour work day, including two hours for instruction in reading and writing.[130]

Together with the exploitation of the children beyond their physical endurance, we see their neglect. Many children had to be admitted to workhouses. The contemporary painter Hogarth has left etchings depicting the child as he made his way through the narrow streets of London, streets infested with dirt and crime. In *Gin Lane* we see a drunken woman carelessly dropping her child from her arms down a long stairway to the street below. Behind her, a man roasts a baby on a spit—a symbol, but nevertheless a reminder of stark realities.

Fielding of Scotland Yard (d. 1750) organized a group of men who became known as "thief takers." A description of the London of this period is given by Hugh Young.

London was a seething underworld in the days of Fielding, and it is known that when he made a raid upon two slum dwellings in Shoreditch, he found nearly a hundred men, women and children crowded into the filthy, reeking rooms; among them were children of five and six years of age who had been taught the nimble art of pocket picking, while those of even more tender years were expert in keeping watch while their parents stole a purse or watch.[131]

Sir Patrick Hastings, in a historical survey of legal cases, has called attention to the story of a child which fits the patterns here described.[132] A boy, born in 1715 of an English lord, was two years old when his parents separated. As was the custom, he stayed with his father, who shortly thereafter took on a young mistress. The woman, in part through her hatred of the child and partly because of her greed for money, had him removed from his good public school when he was seven. So far, there is nothing unusual about the story. But the commentator adds that the child was simply left wandering in the streets, "living upon the charity of anyone who was kind enough to befriend him." Apparently no law would protect this child from being thrown out of his home; no constable appeared to bring charges against the parents. His father died when he was twelve, and four months later he was kidnapped and sold as a slave for the American trade. For thirteen years he attempted to tell his story, which no one believed. He finally succeeded in convincing representatives of the English and the American governments of the veracity of his tale and following this was repatriated and his vindication achieved. Unbelievable as it is to the modern mind that a young boy could for five and a half years live on the streets as a vagrant, without the protection of family or society, it did take place. And we know that this sorry tale was far from unique.

NINETEENTH CENTURY

England. It is a small step and little change from the eighteenth to the nineteenth century, as we pursue our subject. Toward the middle of the eighteenth century the institution of the Foundling Hospital marked a new attitude toward the preservation of the infant's life. Previously boarded out under "wretched conditions," those infants who had survived through the first few months were admitted to the Foundling Hospital, which boasted enlightened care. Artificial feeding, unfortunately under unhygienic conditions, was applied there, and it is reported that mortality was three times as high among the artificially fed as among the breast-fed babies.[133]

Infant mortality was still high; and we learn that in England and Wales between the years 1881-1890 out of every thousand children born annually, one hundred and forty-two died before reaching the age of twelve months.[134]

It is not possible to compare these figures with the mortality of previous years, but we can assume that during the nineteenth century the mortality rate was reduced—possibly to a considerable degree.

It is clear that many children were neglected for a variety of reasons, and that very little or no protection was afforded them by society. We read that in the six years from 1870 to 1877 the school board had taken off the streets of London "8,508 homeless, lawless, and destitute children."[135]

Dickens' novels are rich in illustrations of a child's life in this time: *Oliver Twist* and *The Pickwick Papers* among others. Oliver Twist, born in a workhouse, was "farmed out" with twenty or thirty other "juvenile offenders against the poor laws." Ill fed, ill clothed, working long hours at a coffin maker's, he lived in a damp and dark stone cellar.

Many cruel invectives were hurled at him for being a parish child, and his experiences were probably typical of the majority of parish children. Lessons in pickpocketing, begging, and other expedient ways were part and parcel of the life of underprivileged children of the time. Astute criminals roaming the London streets were all too ready to instruct the young in the more devious ways of making a quick shilling. These children, either neglected by their parents or just out to steal, gathered in gangs, becoming inmates of "flash houses." In two hundred or so of these houses youths of both sexes gathered, about six thousand in number. They were in contact with hardened criminals, in whose path the younger children soon followed.[136] We see a similarity between these and the gangs of today: leadership and hero worship in a set-up of criminal activities.

How common imprisonment of children was, we do not know. However, for the year 1816 we have the figure of three thousand children as prisoners in various London jails. Of these three thousand, all under twenty, almost half were under seventeen.[137] How they were treated once they reached prison we know, for instance, from Oscar Wilde's pamphlet on the subject.[138] A kind warden was dismissed for having given extra food (biscuits) to a child. While most indignant about the treatment of the young prisoners, Wilde tends to put the responsibility on the social system rather than the wardens themselves.

> To shut up a child in a dimly-lit cell for twenty-three hours out of the twenty-four is an example of the cruelty of stupidity—Most warders are very fond of children—But the system prohibits them from rendering the child any assistance.[139]

Very young children were apparently admitted at Reading Gaol for such minor offences as poaching rabbits. To be sure, such an offence in the previous century would have led a child straight to the gallows, but prison life still held no promise of humane treatment.

> The cruelty that is practiced by day and night on children in English prisons is incredible, except to those who have witnessed it and are aware of the brutality of the system.[140]

One boy of thirteen, caught stealing a watch and chain from a chamber in the Temple, was sentenced to death.[141]

The hulks provided an added refinement to the penal art. On these floating prisons, plying the trade to Gibraltar and other ports, young boys were confined with tough criminals. One record of the time provides revealing figures.[142] On one of the hulks were "one child of two, two of twelve, four boys of fourteen, four of fifteen, and altogether twenty persons less than sixteen years old." A special hulk, the *Euryalus*, was reserved, it seems, for boys only. Some children were so young that they could scarcely get into their own clothes. Here, as well as in prisons, the government placed "a number of natural and neglected babies and children."

Child employment took on magnitude with the development of industry. A certain factory owner reported before a House of Lords committee in 1817 that he did not employ children under ten, a noteworthy progress. But it was not until the beginning of the twentieth century that child labor came officially to an end. Children working in the country on farms were in some ways more fortunate, although they hardly worked less than the child population engaged in factory labor.[143]

France. Education in France gradually extended to the masses, and by 1882 compulsory education was established. And it is indeed at the end of the nineteenth century that the psychologists Binet and Simon did psychometric studies of children in public schools, the results of which were published in 1905. They were to become widely known, and the psychometric tests evolved from them are still in use with some modification. By the Guizot law a school was estab-

95

lished in each community where all but poor children were expected to pay a fee.[144] According to Guerard, girls enjoyed the same privileges at a later date (1850).

With the spreading of industrialization, women began to work outside of their homes. In 1844 Firmin Marbeau created the day nursery in the belief that high mortality of children under two was "due to the absence of their working mothers."[145] Thus the need of the young child for its mother was perceived in its relation to a phenomenon generally attributed to physical causes.

Discipline had considerably softened and prohibition of corporal punishment was officially sanctioned with the institution of compulsory education. The family had become smaller, and greater value was now placed on each child. The infant was usually reared by a simple peasant girl who was expected to give a blind and time-absorbing devotion. The child of the poor was kept very close to the mother and nurtured by her. Only in the case of working mothers were babies farmed out to nurses in the country.[146] The importance of the mother or mother-substitute during the early years of childhood came into its own.

The smallness of the family and the importance given each child fostered over-indulgent attitudes on the part of parents. Of this we are told by reputable contemporary historians. Another side of the treatment of children, however, is brought out by laws which appeared at this time. In 1911 several reports on children working at night in glass works were published in Germany as well as in France. They indicate that, although children were compelled to attend school by day, they could also be used for factory work at night. In one of these reports[147] the author's object was to put pressure on the legislature in order to reduce the number of children used as blowers in glass works, though not remove them entirely from these destructive occupations. As we can see, the utilization of the child was still in force, and the Law of the Twelve Tables still influenced customs, even though it had lost its official standing and dropped its overt viciousness.

The apparent submissiveness of children rendered easy the marriages of convenience which were then the rule, according to the historians Barker and Edwards.[148, 149] There is

96

also evidence that, while the child got more affection and warmth from his parents, he was still under their close domination. It is difficult from sources consulted to reconstruct the parent-child relationship and the emotional disturbances which may have arisen in the family set-up.

Causes of the women's rebellion which was to come at the beginning of the twentieth century may be seen in the excessive domination of parents and the overpowering assumption of responsibility for their children, in particular for their daughters. Some signs of rebellion are seen elsewhere. The problem of "insubordinate" children (comparable to the juvenile delinquents of today) took on a magnitude which brought forth laws for the creation of special centers where children in difficulties with society were to be admitted. At first (1842) a special department within the jail was circumscribed, and it was not until 1850 that institutions admitting only children were opened.[150]

Let us not be deluded about the modicum of insight afforded children. We find in Bonzon a chapter covering this period, 1850-1890, in which just about all psychiatric problems are covered under the following heading: *"L'enfance insoumise et coupable."*[151] There were no other nuances. A child who departed from established behavior patterns was fitted into one of two categories—the insubordinate or the guilty—the latter a clear reminder of the Middle Ages' "original sin."

America. Calhoun's second volume is aptly titled *The Emancipation of the Child.* "In a society whose population is small as compared with available resources, children always occupy an important position. . . ."[152] It is ironical that, in a large measure, it was owing to his economic usefulness that the child rose in status to heights heretofore unknown, and which could not have been anticipated. There was a compactness and a unity in the pioneer family which are lacking in contemporary families in the western world. Pioneer women generally nursed their own children, in part because of the absence of medical facilities, according to Calhoun. Undoubtedly, the dangers from the outside which were threatening to the family also contributed to its closeness and in binding its members to one another.

Another trend is evident: a degree of freedom accorded the child—a trend without parallel in the western world. The child takes on importance in the eyes of the adult, and we find a comment in Calhoun which is significant of this development.

An educational journal of 1833 contains an interesting description of the new cult of childhood. The attention furnished now on children forms an interesting feature of the day. An interest seems to be rekindling, analogous to that which animated the ancient philosophers.[153]

The emancipation of the child is commented upon by all observers, each from his own point of view. Naumann in his *Nord Amerika*, 1848, comments that, if a father has been too severe with his son, the latter can go to the Justice of the Peace to have his father punished.[154] Fine or prison was the usual penalty.

It is obvious that the rules applying to behavior have greatly mellowed, and that efforts are made at an understanding of children's needs and of their specific ways of reacting to their environment.

An educational journal in 1833 recorded that "Mothers have derived new ideas of education, and entered with increased intelligence and zeal into the discharge of their duties. . . . The infant school has become an assistant, an observatory to the mother; and the season of infancy and childhood, a period of progress and enjoyment."[155]

Visitors from the Old World were voluble in their criticism of the new freedom accorded children. As early as 1807 a distressed foreigner wrote,

One of the greatest evils of a Republican form of government is a loss . . . of subordination in society . . . Boys assume the air of full grown coxcombs. This is not to be wondered at, when most parents make it a principle never to check those ungovernable passions that are born with us, or to correct the growing vices of their children.[156]

An Englishwoman in 1848 comments that the unhappy state of affairs in America was not duplicated in her country.

The indulgence which parents in the United States permit to their children is not seen in England; the child is too early his own master; as soon as he can sit at table he chooses his own food, and as soon as he can speak argues with his parents on the propriety or impropriety of their directions.[157]

Some Americans are in disagreement with the excess of freedom granted children. One writer says,

Strictly speaking there is no such thing as social subordination in the United States. Parents have no command over their children. . . . Owing perhaps to the very popular nature of our institutions, the American children are seldom taught that profound reverence for, and strict obedience to their parents, which are at once the basis of domestic comfort and of the welfare of the children themselves.[158]

The *Ladies' Repository* placed the blame on the "fearful decline in family religion."

Certain accounts must admit of exaggeration. We read in a labor newspaper of the time, the daily *Man* of March 21, 1834, the piece entitled "A Modern Catechism Adapted to the Times:"

Who is the oldest man? The lad of fourteen who struts and swaggers and smokes his cigar, and drinks rum; treads on the toes of his grandfather, swears at his mother and sister, and vows that he will run away and leave the 'old man' if he will not let him have more cash.[159]

The freedom and, at times, indulgence of American children does not, however, complete our picture of their life. Darker colors filled in the gaps. It was hardly an over-indulgent attitude on the part of adults that led a fourteen-year-old boy from New Jersey to the following fate in 1829. This crime is not stated, but we know that he was held in prison with a group of hardened criminals.

The boy, being undersized, was small enough to crawl through the grating in the prison doors. Therefore the prison officials put on him an iron yoke into which his head was placed and to which his arms were fastened in such a way as to keep his arms extended some twenty inches apart on a level with his shoulders.[160]

Rare instances notwithstanding, it is clear that radical changes have taken place in the status of the child in family and society. In the long historical view of this evolution the changes are so extreme that they can be qualified as revolutionary. Bold as it may seem, one feels justified in speaking of an *American Child Revolution*. Little wonder that so much confusion has resulted in the field of child psychology. Guilt feelings must weigh heavily on generation after generation. It was a sudden, momentous, almost cataclysmic upheaval that took place at the beginning of the nineteenth century in America in the "freeing" of the child. Actually, if we are to trust contemporaneous writings, children were freeing themselves rather than being freed. Rebellion came first, and the freedom was contingent upon the rebellion. While knowledge of child psychology has since grown steadily, the attitudes of parents and of society toward the child have not shown the same steadiness. Vacillations and inconsistencies in the attitudes of parents and society toward the child stem from the tearing apart of family and social structure brought on by the American Child Revolution.

Part Three

THE EMOTIONALLY
HEALTHY CHILD

GENERAL CONSIDERATIONS

The concept of the emotionally healthy child is even more recent than its counterpart, the emotionally disturbed child. The end of the nineteenth and the beginning of the twentieth century mark the advent of an interest in the child as such. Psychological studies of the child are permeated at first with the contrast between normal and abnormal behavior with stress on and precedence of "abnormality."

THE NORMAL CHILD
(Or Rather, Emotionally Healthy Child)

Norms Are Variable. Defining the normal child obviously must be fraught with considerable difficulties, since we so seldom find a definition of the concept in psychiatric textbooks, whether applied to child or adult. As it is generally used, the concept is based on a knowledge of the *norms*. These *norms* are determined through statistical evaluations of large numbers of individuals. It is immediately clear that they do not take into account the dynamics of behavior. Probably, the dynamics of behavior will always elude statistics.

There are those writers who are fond of saying that "there is no such thing as a normal child." They point out that neurotic manifestations can be found in the normal individual, to whom they refer as "so-called normal." Again, we see in this point of view how "normality" is elusive and relative, and how degrees and subtle shadings challenge classifications of human behavior.

To some writers the concept of normality calls immediately for its opposite. We find Menninger indignant over the use of this concept, because of the implication of opposites that it carries.

> The adjuration to be "normal" seems shockingly repellent to me; I see neither hope nor comfort in sinking to that low level. I think it is ignorance that makes people think of abnormality only with horror and allows them to remain undismayed at the proximity of "normal" to average and mediocre. For surely anyone who achieves anything is, *a priori,* abnormal. . . .[1]

Normal behavior, which is not necessarily equivalent to average and mediocre, is more often than not described in a negative way, i.e., described for what it is not: lack of conflict, absence of anxiety, and the like.

The difficulties in approaching the concept of the normal individual are born of the fact that normality is protean, that there is not one clear-cut, fixed frame of reference, but rather a multiplicity of modes which have a common basis. Place and time, influence of cultures and accepted forms of behavior in these cultures are some of the variants. In a brilliant little book, *More About Psychiatry,* Carl Binger has dramatically illustrated the point of variations in space. What would be "normal behavior" in India may be frankly pathological in our society.

Dr. Binger asks us to project the following situation. A well-to-do, established lawyer, Mr. Crawford, leaves his home as usual for work one morning, but on the way discards his coat, his jacket, his shoes, and buys a tin cup. Arriving at his office building, he sits cross-legged in front of it, holding his cup and lost in thought. Thus he remains until five o'clock, when a policeman notices him and hustles him off to Bellevue. And Dr. Binger adds,

Suppose that Crawford's name had been Swamarami, and his skin not sallow white but a rich brown, and that he had taken off his jewelled turban and his silk robes and seated himself under a banyan tree; who would have been considered abnormal, the holy man or the constable who had arrested him?[2]

A man could be worshipped in India for the same behavior which in New York City would send him promptly to a state hospital. What is normal behavior in a multi-million industrial city would appear very odd in a native African village—and vice versa.

Variations in time are illustrated in the recent book by Margaret Mead, *New Lives for Old*. After twenty-five years, she returned to Manus and reported her observations on the great changes which had taken place in this short span of time. The leap had been over centuries in a matter of an almost negligible number of years. In examining her purposes and methods for this project she refers to the "sheer detective work of finding out what had 'really happened' to transform this small cluster of stone-age head-hunters into a community asking for a place in the modern world. . . ."[3]

Again, what is in Manus considered normal behavior in 1953 would not have been thus considered in 1928, since such profound modifications have taken place in that interval. The revamping of responsibilities and work interrelations within the family is illustrated by many of Mead's observations. Take, for instance, the position of the adolescent boys, who are called upon to do more "productive" work than they did twenty-five years past. With the obligation also to attend school, they experience conflict within themselves as well as with their parents. Similarly, the position of women has shifted to activities which were formerly carried out by men.

In addition to cultural patterns which, as we have briefly seen, vary in time and space, other factors play a role, such as sex, age, level of maturation, and even, to a degree, profession. The man on the assembly line cannot permit himself any daydreaming, whereas to the poet it amounts to a creative need.

What Is an Emotionally Healthy Child? A first glance at an emotionally healthy child and you know that he is comfortable with himself, his family, and his social group, and that they, in turn, are comfortable with him. This inner comfort and two-way communication are complex and want elaboration.

The inner contentment proceeds from a sense of security, a sense of being loved and wanted. If this child can accept love, he can also give it in all of its positive expressions and without anxiety about the giving. While he needs human companionship at his level of maturation, he can also for varying periods find satisfaction within himself and accept solitude as a chance for self-realization. These fantasying periods notwithstanding, he is at all times in affective contact with his milieu. He is capable of reacting with anxiety to situations that threaten him; and he attempts to deal with them, provided they are not in fact overwhelming, with a proportionate defensive approach. He can be aggressive and angry when the need is required, principally in defending his own integrity, but he has accepted the prohibitions imposed by his social milieu, and his anger is commensurate with the stimulus that caused it. He functions to the full capacity of his native endowments at his maturation level. His creativeness is a result of the full expression of his abilities without block, or, to the contrary, of an excessive urge to do for the sake exclusively of doing. His activities are purposeful and at his maturation level, but he also can enjoy leisure or play between periods of activity. However distinctive and highly individualized the symbolism of his language and actions may be, it is still intelligible to others.

This admittedly sketchy description should not create the impression of a static condition. On a core of oneness and sameness there is a quality of flexibility and fluctuation in reaction to internal as well as external stimuli. This individual is clearly a part of his social group and conforming to its demands. However, he is not lost as a mere number in this social group. His individuation and uniqueness stamp him as differentiated from all others, yet predictable.

106

Factors Influencing the Formation of Character. Three sets of factors are known to influence the formation of character: heredity, constitution, and environment.

The term "hereditary characteristics" should be strictly confined to those characteristics which are transmitted through the genes. Debates have been raging, and still are, on the question of heredity versus environment. There is fairly general agreement that physiological and morphological characteristics are genetically transmitted, but even the more extensively studied problem of congenital mental deficiency has its protagonists and antagonists. Kanner,[4] quoting various sources, points out the "considerable statistical discrepancies." He tells us, for instance, that the variations of assumed inheritance of deficiency range from twenty-nine per cent (Penrose) to ninety per cent (Hollingworth).

When it comes to psychological makeup, the picture is still more confusing. We do not refer here to loose language as reflected in such statements as "he has inherited his uncle's or his mother's happy (or cranky) disposition," a transmission which could hardly be operated through the genes.

In the first place, how can the earliest environmental influences be isolated from hereditary influences, since the parents, who are the agents for hereditary transmission, are also, at first entirely and later to a large extent, the child's environment? The problem could be solved only under research conditions which would make it possible to dissociate the two sets of influences: for instance, careful studies of the antecedents of actual parents of children who are adopted at birth, with comparative studies of the antecedents of their adoptive parents and of the children themselves.

Numerous clinical observations point to the importance of parents or parent-substitutes as the earliest environment of the child. It is common to find that a child adopted in a family has, over a period of years, taken on not only psychological features but physical ones as well, the latter referring particularly to facial structure and expression. Granted, agencies in placing children for adoption take great pains to match religion, stock, ages, and social status. Nevertheless, the matching is only grossly approximate and could not account for finer similarities.

107

A known sociological fact also challenges the stand of heredity. Large numbers of immigrants from Central and Northern Europe with physiological and morphological characteristics outstandingly in contrast with the modern American body-type have, in the course of one generation (sometimes two), produced this very American body-type. This means a transition from short, pyknic body types to the long, muscular type. Psychological characteristics are also in striking contrast with those of the earlier generations, a fact often cited as a basis for conflict between two successive generations.

Constitution refers to the physical makeup and the functional patterns (physiological and intellectual) which are present at birth. Differences in constitutional endowments and patterns are sometimes very conspicuous within a family of several children. Heredity plays a part; so do prenatal conditions which, to date, have not been satisfactorily studied. Of these prenatal conditions the physical and emotional state of the mother during pregnancy may be foremost.

The earliest environment of the infant is its mother, and during the formative years it is primarily its family. Modern studies are emphasizing more and more the role of these influences on the formation of character.

Some Considerations Relating to Emotional Development. Since the brilliant discoveries by Freud, light has been thrown on the emotional development of the child. This especially pertains to infantile sexuality as the basis for healthy psychosexual adult adjustment.

Five periods will be considered in the span of life which extends from birth to adulthood:

> the first year of life;
> one to three years;
> three to six years;
> six to thirteen years;
> thirteen to eighteen years.

The first three periods, i.e., from birth to six, are not only the periods of greatest change, but they are also the periods in which the changes are most meaningful and actually form the foundation of the adult personality. These are the formative years. The five periods should be considered arbitrary only in so far as they are divided into clear-cut delineation for purposes of convenience. Nevertheless, they correspond roughly to the greatest and most meaningful physical changes, although there is no cause-effect determination. Rather, there is an interplay and interrelationship between these two sets of factors.

To illustrate: a child who for physical reasons does not learn to walk until three years, whereas the normal is between twelve and fifteen months, is likely to be held at an earlier level of emotional maturity, since the physical lag will retard his exploration of and contact with the outside physical world. Similarly, the fact that a girl has her menstrual onset at sixteen, instead of the more usual age of twelve, is likely to influence social and emotional growth.

One more point to be emphasized is that the changes take place in a movement of constant fluctuation with forward trend and not on a fixed, straight, and immutable line. This point cannot be emphasized enough. In recent years mothers have enjoyed the privilege, denied previous generations, of a wealth of literature on the growth and care of children. The information has been helpful to be sure, but it has also created a form of slavery to standards and schedules. This is often revealed when mothers are asked to give an account of their children's early years, whether the latter be free from emotional disturbances or not: as, for instance, during registration in some progressive school or in application for treatment. "He walked at twelve and a half months just like the book said he should. . . . I was very upset because she didn't start to talk until two years and the book emphatically said that she should have uttered single words between twelve and fifteen months. . . . He is definitely a 'Book' baby."

The First Year of Life. The life of an individual begins officially at the moment of birth but is determined to some extent before that moment. This refers particularly to prenatal influences which have been but little investigated. One recent study, not published to date, bears on the point. In a group of fourteen women observed during and after pregnancy, A. E. Hamilton studied the relation between the emotional and the physical state during pregnancy.[5] According to this writer, women who shared love and sexual satisfaction with their husbands, who enjoyed the emotional support of their husbands, found pregnancy a satisfactory experience both physically and emotionally. The other women suffered discomfort, nausea, obsessive fears, etc. When the time for labor approached, women who were emotionally immature (frigidity, sexually anxious, etc.) showed ambivalent feelings in anticipation of delivery, whereas women with a secure emotional background looked forward to labor.

The ability to breast-feed depended similarly on the emotional support these women had had from their husbands and on their freedom from anxiety about sex. For the seven women who had a good sexual-emotional adjustment, breast feeding was an enjoyable experience. Only one of the others was able to breast-feed her baby satisfactorily and with pleasure. Limited in its scope, this study points to certain trends which need further and wider investigation. At any rate, there is no need to emphasize the close relation between the well-being of the mother, pre- and post-delivery, and the well-being of the infant at birth.

During the period of gestation, the child has grown in a state of symbiosis with the mother. Symbiosis is medically defined as "the living together or close association of two dissimilar organisms." The embryo is in a state of physical dependence which is absolute and on which its life depends. It lives, in fact, as if the total maternal organism had taken on a new internal organ and function. Far from being destructive to the psycho-biological balance of the mother, it generally adds a feeling of satisfaction and emotional richness which many mothers-to-be are likely to report: "I was never so well as during my pregnancy." Certain pathological conditions, such as tuberculosis or heart disease, and various neurotic states, of course, alter this picture.

The physiological milieu of the embryo presents definite characteristics. The fetus is not only in absolute dependence on the mother for nourishment, minerals, oxygen, etc., which are essential to its growth, but its milieu is shock-proof and

110

free from external stimuli (except for rare traumatic experiences). The temperature is constant and variations are at a minimum. All the necessary chemical substances for the fetus' growth are provided in an entirely passive way from the placenta. Organs of the fetus which will be called upon to function in post-uterine stages are not only in abeyance, but some of them are not fully developed. This refers particularly to the respiratory organs and the gastro-intestinal tract. Circulation follows a pattern which in relation to post-natal life is only temporary and must be redirected. The central nervous system is undeveloped, and myelinization of nervous tracts is not only incomplete at birth but for some of them will not be completed for several years. Monakow and Mourgue divide neurological development into seven phases ranging from the simplest functions shortly after birth—sucking etc.—to the most complex "terminal growth" at five to ten years, when the coordination and adaptation in space and time of motor and sensory function are achieved.[6]

At the moment of birth the child enters abruptly a world which is in direct contrast with these uniform and stable conditions. The psychological effect of this complete reversal has been described by Freud and emphasized by Rank as the first anxiety-reaction in the human being.[7, 8] Normally, the child is not overwhelmed by the anxiety which is necessarily created by this sudden disruption of his physical tranquility. However, certain birth conditions, prolonged or in any way traumatic to the infant, may modify the capacity of the small body to deal with them. "A predisposition to anxiety" may thus be created which will in later years influence the child's defenses against anxiety.[9, 10]

At birth the child is completely helpless, dependent, and incomplete. This absolute dependence continues for several months and its continuance is the *sine qua non* for survival for a long period to come. As much as is possible, the uniformity of conditions existing in intra-uterine life must be preserved, with changes introduced gradually.

Perhaps no other writer has given a more enlightening, inclusive, and sensitive description of the infant's physical and emotional needs than Margaret Ribble in *The Rights of Infants*. Her conclusions are based on sound physiological ob-

111

servation which has not heretofore been tied up with the infant's emotional needs.

In utero the fetus relies for sustenance entirely on the placenta. Respiration and gastro-intestinal function have not been established in the pattern of their ultimate destination, even though the organs are developed and in abeyance. Neither does circulation follow the functional patterns which are found after birth and must, of necessity, be then initiated. Ribble reminds us that the animal (particularly the mammal) mother is able to help its newborn through continuous body contact, body warmth, skin stimulation (licking), and sustaining food (breast milk). The total nervous system is markedly undeveloped.

Breathing at birth—and this because it is an entirely nascent function—is inadequate, tentative, and erratic. These characteristics would apply to any function which is in the process of being established with organs which have not previously served toward their ultimate purpose.

Oxygen which throughout the intra-uterine life has been brought to the fetus solely by way of the placental blood must now be sucked in through the lungs. There is thus a complex readjustment of the organs involved in prenatal and postnatal breathing.

In addition, there is an overlapping of prenatal and postnatal functions. For instance, the diaphragm is used temporarily after birth as a suction pump drawing oxygenated blood from the liver. This was the diaphragm's function during intra-uterine life, and although it becomes eventually unnecessary, it is still present for a short period after birth.

The baby, then, is physiologically unprepared to cope efficiently with his body's great need for oxygen during the first month of life. His proper brain development rests upon the fulfillment of this need, for the brain at birth is in an undeveloped state and needs large supplies of oxygen for its normal growth. Equally dependent on breathing is speech. Not until normal breathing has been established will the baby attempt to vocalize. How can an adequate oxygen supply be taken in, when his respiration is still functioning somewhat in reverse order? The lungs and chest must develop strength. The diaphragm must reverse its former function.

It seems at first glance far-fetched to say that mothering can have any effect on respiration. But on closer examination of the reactions of the newborn we find that this is true. Cuddling, fondling and all body contact give the infant the stimulation needed to promote steady, deep respiration. His breathing in its earliest stages depends largely on his mother's touch. Here we have the first instance of the close relationship between the physical and emotional needs of the infant. We will find as we continue that these needs are inseparable.

It is commonly thought that the infant's "all-absorbing activity," sucking, is single-purposed, motivated only by the need to get food. But the needs, psychological as well as physiological, fulfilled by sucking are many. It provides the infant with his first contact with the outer world, his first sense of pleasure and security. Hospital observation has brought out that when infants were deprived of sucking, except as a means of taking in food, they compensated by thumb-sucking. The work of David Levy on sucking deprivation and its destructive effects is too well known to need elaboration.[11]

Sucking is instinctive. Some infants are born sucking their fingers. The development of the embryo tells much about the story of the importance of sucking. The mouth is fundamentally connected with touch, as embryological studies show, for it develops from skin which folds in to form a pouch. Only on the sixth week of fetal growth does the hard palate start to develop, thus separating the mouth into a cavity for eating and breathing. The tongue, at first closely connected with the brain, fulfills various functions in the growth of the fetus. It is probable that, very early, its pumping action supplies blood to the brain. By the seventh month it provides the fetus with the first sensations of touch through back-and-forth motion over the hard palate. The tongue's subsequent relation to speech is foreseen in its close connection with the brain via cranial nerves.

Although the infant is born with the sucking reflex, it may be necessary to stimulate this reflex at birth. This can be done by closing the infant's mouth around his mother's breast and moving his chin in a rhythmic sucking motion. So does Ribble view the mother's help to her infant when sucking is insufficient.

The mother plays an all-important role in thus stimulating a reflex basic to certain emotional and physical adjustment. Through this contact with the outer world, he is to develop a sense of security and pleasure. Only after the sucking need has diminished, normally toward the end of the fourth month, will he begin to experiment with vocalization and with other approaches to his surroundings, such as grasping with his hands and biting. Sucking also aids in the development of breathing. It adds to body alertness and improved muscle tone. In the same way is circulation stimulated.

By the second month of life, sucking becomes related to the functions of seeing and hearing. The infant in its mother's arms at this time begins to respond with his eyes, seemingly staring intently at his mother's face. At this time the sound of her voice can give him added security. This is the time, too, when the smile appears. In these ways the growing awareness and development of the baby depend much on the fulfillment of the need to suck, a need which can be fulfilled by the mother's close body contact with her child, by the sense of security and well-being which this contact affords the child. It is through such closeness with the mother that the baby first senses love, the first stage of what later becomes a complex emotion. In later years this will be the foundation of his ability to give and receive love.

There are other important physical-psychological contacts of mother and infant which further the latter's growth and adjustment. Ribble groups certain of these under the category of "learning to feel."

The mother again is called upon to offer the stimulus to promote the infant's development. There is the skin stimulus, aiding both circulation and reflex activities. Many babies would go without this stimulus altogether were it not that their mothers or nurses were concerned with strict cleanliness and administered daily baths and rubbings.

The dog and the cat with their litters know instinctively the importance of this contact between mother and offspring. The bitch licks her puppies, the cat her kittens. We are inclined to think of this as a concern for cleanliness. But, as

Ribble reports young puppies bred in Cornell University laboratories have died under experimental conditions because they were deprived of licking.

The mother is again instrumental in the well-being of her baby in helping him establish his sense of position—his physical relation to space. In the uterus he had spatial security. His neo-natal world is vastly different and frightening. The danger of falling seems always at hand. We think of the rocking chair and the cradle as old-fashioned, and not many years ago mothers were warned about jiggling and rocking their babies. But the motion of the cradle, the motion of rocking in a mother's arms can help the infant regain his sense of security in relation to the space around him. The closeness of his mother's body, the sound of her voice, and the rhythmic motion are all necessary to the baby, if he is eventually to develop confidence and self-reliance.

It is not possible for a baby to get his bearings in space. It is also difficult for him to become accustomed to sounds. Sudden loud noise is a violent shock to the infant. He needs help to get used to the sounds around him. This help can come best from his mother, from the gentle tones of her voice, from the soothing and rhythmic lullaby she sings as she holds and rocks him. With her help, sound can become a pleasure, instead of a shocking experience.

There can, of course, be an overdose of any or all of these stimuli. The baby reacts with anxiety to deprivation, he so reacts as well to over-stimulation. Too-frequent diapering and the skin stimulation it entails may lead the baby to place too much importance on one area of his body, associating it with a means of getting pleasure and attention. Needless to say, great difficulties can follow. Or a baby can be rocked too often and too long. He may become over-dependent, not being given the chance to try out his muscles on his own. But there can be no mistake, if the mother is close to her baby and aware of his reactions. He will make known his developing needs. Her loving response to these needs cannot be far wrong.

We are prone to take for granted that the baby sleeps a deep and natural sleep from the day of birth on. Actually, his first weeks of sleep are a kind of hibernation, a semi-consciousness, for the newborn has neither the oxygen supply nor the brain development to engage in any mental activity. For the first month his waking and sleeping hours are much alike. He has not yet developed the rhythm of sleep, the rhythm of activity followed by rest.

Sleep depends on activity, for it is made necessary by activity. The baby sleeps after stimulation. And the mother again provides stimulus for the very young infant, thus starting him on a regular rhythmic pattern of activity and rest.

Following the certain sensory satisfactions, such as eating, the baby is ready for sleep. Then it is that his mother can hold him in her arms, offering him the security of her presence, perhaps rocking him to sleep. This will fulfill many needs. Besides providing the stimulation that will lead to sleep, and the satisfaction of his mother's presence, it will help him in adjusting to his surroundings, to his self-awareness and his awareness of position in space. Sleep, as we know from the young child, can be a very frightening experience, an abandonment of the consciousness to the unknown, a manner of death. The child's feeling is reflected in the familiar prayer, quoted by Ribble.

> Now I lay me down to sleep,
> I pray the Lord my soul to keep.
> If I should die before I wake,
> I pray the Lord my soul to take.

A mother's presence, her soothing voice can provide the sense of security needed at this time.

Without this attention before sleep, without the gentle rocking of the cradle or his mother's arms, the baby will have to provide his own stimulus. And the only way he can do that at this time is by sucking his thumb (later rocking is used in the same way). It hardly need be said that this can be the beginning of a habit that is very difficult to give up.

A baby suffers from lack of stimulation. At this point let us be mindful of the destructive manifestation of hospitalism described by Spitz,[12] and of the still more extreme forms found in the marasmus of the historical past, not too distant as well as very remote. But the baby can also have too much stimulation. He develops quickly, his needs change, and he gradually becomes more and more self-reliant. The mother should recognize this growing readiness for independence. And she must remember that the stimulation she offers her baby is not an end in itself but only a means to initiate the baby's own development, to help him in realizing himself and his relation to the external world.

At the end of the first year the infant has achieved a higher level of maturation which is evident in all spheres. He has reached a small degree of physical independence from his mother, in particular with his first steps. This partial physical independence he has gained through his mother, as elaborated earlier. He has become aware of the world outside himself through the very alternating of having and not having his mother. In a very small way he has begun to communicate with the outside world, mainly his mother, and the sounds that he is now producing have the beginning of purpose and meaning. Through the security that his mother in fulfilling his needs has been able, fully or not, to give him, his emotional reactions already have a stamp of individuality, in particular his way of reacting to frustrations. He already has a personality of his own.

A decade or two ago the young child would not have been thought of as having a personality. Again we are indebted to Ribble for the enlightenment given in her book of the very title *The Personality of the Young Child*. The enormous importance of the first year of life as a basis for later emotional adjustment, the role played by the mother-infant relationship during that first year—these are very recent acquisitions. To Spitz we are also indebted for further understanding of the significance of the mother to her infant and his later emotional stability. In several articles which will be discussed under the subject of emotional disturbances, he has reported observations on infants who were deprived of their mothers and on the resulting destructive effects on the child's total development.

The infant's life is activated by the need to fulfill his instinctual urges. The degree of satisfaction obtained in fulfilling these urges (he is obviously at this time all instinct, no ego, no superego) has a significance in giving a direction to his future development. In this connection the psychological impact of the infant's oral dependency is paramount. In Freudian terminology this period of life is accordingly described as the oral phase. We have seen that the link between the infant and his mother is the source of the child's awareness of himself and his relation to the outside world in its most primitive form. It is in this respect as well as the satisfaction of physical requirements that mothering constitutes a vital need of the infant.

While it is not possible quantitatively to evaluate the importance of each of the three periods aggregating to the formative years (birth to six), the importance of the first year of life cannot be overemphasized. Indeed, in some severe emotional disturbances such as early infantile autism, this importance stands out in glaring relief.

One to Three Years. The next two years have an importance of their own, and this because some developments take place which have a direct bearing on the formation of character. Certain outstanding stages of growth and training are reached in this period, which again is strictly delineated for purposes of convenience only. It is during this period that elimination training takes place and is generally achieved. Speech, while not reaching the complexity found at the adult level, has, nevertheless, all its simple structural elements. Reality testing and ego development (discovery of self and what is not-self), curiosity about self and not-self, all related, are gradually established. Mild anxiety arising from certain dynamics to be elaborated upon, and also from anxious dreams, are normally experienced during this period. Ambivalent feelings (love-hate) are normally exhibited. And finally, aggressiveness with destructive tendencies is part of normal behavior during that stage.

Parents may well have been confused by the varied and often contradictory advice which has been given them through pediatricians or pamphlet literature handed to them during the past quarter of a century. Whatever the method may have been, the mothers have trained their children to habits made necessary by social living. It is well known that excessive demands were made upon the child during the first stage of parent education (early part of twentieth century). Several cases have come to the attention of the writer where the mother stated that she had "begun at birth" the training of her child, meaning by this that the infant was constantly observed, in an attempt to establish the schedule of his elimination. This, in addition, required frequent investigation of the diapers and constant fussing, which does not add to emotional comfort and security but rather the opposite, i.e., a kind of mechanization of the mother-child relationship.

These are very rare exceptions which lead subsequently to severe emotional disturbances. They are of interest, however, as they represent pathological extremes of a tendency which was general in earlier times and still persists to a degree. It was thought that habit formation must begin as early as possible; emotional maturity as well as muscular maturity were not taken into consideration. Tensions, disturbed mother-child relationship, and compulsive ways of behaving, among other disturbances, arose as a result.

In the second phase parent education went to the other extreme. The *laissez-faire* attitude, however, did not mark an improvement. Healthy elimination training is based on an understanding of the physical and emotional readiness of the child. Physical readiness requires neurological and muscular growth which permits function and absence of organic conditions which would interfere with it. Emotional readiness refers essentially to the mother-child relationship.

Elimination training represents the first demands which are made upon the child. Prior to this, the life of the infant has followed this cycle: expression of instinctual urges, satisfaction, and pleasure in receiving satisfaction. We have here the source of the feeling of omnipotence experienced by the infant which gradually subsides during the early childhood years. During elimination training, as pointed out in psychoanalytic writing, the child is giving up something which is precious to him as part of his body. It is easier for him to do what his mother demands of him without tension or negativism, if he feels secure with his mother, her warmth and love having made him feel so.

Neurotic problems, and they are many, which arise from this situation can usually be traced from an unsatisfactory relation between mother and child. The mother may, because of an excessive drive for cleanliness, be tense and insistent. The child needs no vocabulary to sense his mother's feelings. Muscular tensions, tone of voice, and the like are enough. We do not give enough credit to acuteness of sensory perception in the infant. Films taken in the course of a several years' study by Margaret Fries are explicit on the subject. Mothers were studied with their babies in the breast-feeding situation, and the contrast between maternal attitudes and their effects on the nursing infant is very striking. The frustrations of babies in reaction to their mothers' inner tensions were emphatically demonstrated.

Films are not available to reveal the mother-child relationship in the elimination training situation. The emotional climate and its effects on the child are the same. We must recall that the child is not repelled by his excretions. To the contrary, he experiences pleasure in the handling of his excreta, when he has a chance to get at them. He is in no way prepared, therefore, for the dilemma of his mother's openly expressed disgust, if this is manifested. As is known, the smearing of feces is likely to be more persistent, if the mother is compulsively clean and shows a determination to prohibit a—to her—taboo activity. In passing, such mothers are expressing problems of their own with regard to sex and elimination.

Prior to the initiation of elimination training, the mother has been aware of a kind of rhythmicity of excretory functions which is peculiar to her own child. The healthy mother has not been overly preoccupied and unduly active about watching it, but she has some inkling of when it will be easier for the child to perform, and she utilizes this knowledge. The level of maturation of excretory organs must be considered. Obviously, if the nerves activating the muscles which permit the sitting position are not myelinated, the mother cannot expect her child to sit comfortably and urinate.

By the time he has reached one year (beginning at 6 to 8 months) the infant is normally able to sit. However, the standing position, which is required of little boys, cannot be comfortably assumed for voiding until a higher level of nervous maturation is reached with a concomitant stability of the lower limbs established.

120

Although the cortical fibres must be myelinated before voluntary sphincter control can be established, it is possible, but not desirable, to establish training through segmental conditioned reflex.[13] Heavy demands are then made upon immature cortical pathways. The tendency toward personality over-organization and compulsive behavior is amply demonstrated in clinical observations of neurotic individuals whose elimination training was carried out by a compulsive mother.[14]

With the boy, the situation is further complicated by the fact that the boy, unlike the girl, goes through two successive trainings. First, he must learn to void sitting down, then standing up. The latter stage takes place when the child is already a toddler. As a result, there is a well-recognized predominance of boys over girls in so far as enuretic behavior and neurotic problems are concerned. Because of the paramount importance of the mother-child relation, it is fitting that several factors here involved be considered.

A greater complexity of motor attitudes and a further degree of nervous maturation are required to void in a standing position. At this stage there is still a lack of coordination in walking (developmental ataxia), and this is paralleled by a lack of stability in the standing position. In addition, to direct the stream requires that fine manual dexterity be achieved and also requires some manipulation on the part of the mother. Finally, the dissociation between control of urethral and anal centers must be achieved. All these factors tend to increase tensions, if the little boy is not physically ready for the performance demanded of him.

There is also involved here the additional touch stimulation required of the mother (seduction), a factor of no negligible significance. What the small child needs is readiness and support, not stimulation. When the mother has given the emotional support needed, the child goes through this complex phase of elimination training without giving cause for conflict.

Again it must be pointed out that, while landmarks are given with chronological definiteness, development normally shows fluctuations (advances and apparent regressions with over-all progress). The first sounds produced by the infant have no language significance, for we have seen that the cry primarily serves respiration.

It is highly significant that the first stage of communication is not only associated with feeding so that the first phonetic sounds are of the "m" order, involving muscles of the lips and tongue used in sucking, but are also designed to serve in the first communication with the mother, "mum." In this sense, these sounds represent the first verbal contact of the infant with the outside world.

Speech distinguishes man from the animals, not only because of the emission of complex phonetic sounds, but primarily because of the symbolism of his language.

Single words are uttered toward the end of the first year, and it is during the 1 to 3 year period that sentence structure in a simple form becomes instituted. However simple the structure may be, it, nevertheless, achieves a minimal structural organization, which is found in elaborate form at the adult level.

Children show marked variations in the rhythm and pattern of speech development. It is found that, within normal limits, one child will have achieved basic structural language at two years, whereas another will not reach that level until four. The first one is precocious, the second is somewhere around the upper limit, but both levels represent normal growth. By basic structural language is meant the minimal structural organization found in the correct use of subject, verb, object ("Daddy come home. . . . Mommy cook dinner").

Toward the end of the 1 to 3 year period the child has a tendency either to repeat syllables or to block on some syllables. This frequently arouses anxiety in the parents, who, in some cases, work with determination at "correcting" what they consider a defect. However, this *developmental stutter* is a normal phenomenon, due to the fact that the child thinks faster than his organs of phonation, still biologically immature, would permit him to speak.

As indicated in an earlier study, the speech function is dependent upon two fundamental requirements, the desire to speak and the means of speaking.[15] In order to be able to communicate with the environment the child must first have the desire to do so. The desire to speak obviously depends upon affective factors—it is not uncommon to find young children with a history of frustrations and unhappy situations presenting also a history of delayed speech development. Child psychiatrists are also familiar with the temporary speech regressions which are associated with psychic traumata in early childhood. The means of speaking depends on three basic requirements: a normally functioning intelligence, an adequate auditory system, and adequate organs of expression for phonation and articulation of vocal sounds.

EGO DEVELOPMENT:

During the first year of life the infant has gradually acquired a somewhat fragmentary awareness of the physical self. During the period under discussion, the child develops a realization of self, and ego development takes place. As is well known, the main function of the ego, the core of the personality, is reality testing. This is reflected in the language phase now under consideration. The realization of self (I—not-I, self—not-self) is mirrored in language forms which are familiar to all of us. This is the period in which the child, echoing his mother, refers to himself in the second person ("you go to sleep") or in the third person ("he is naughty"). A regression to these earlier forms is common in some severe emotional disturbances such as schizophrenia. It is further noted that as the patient improves or recovers, his regained realization of self is mirrored in the return of the "I" form.

The realization of self in the young child during this period is again aided by the emotional security his mother can give him. If his relationship with his mother is ungratifying and fraught with frustrations, the ego development will show disturbances of varying severity. While these disturbances may not be conspicuous at the time, or even be suspected, repercussions on later personality development may be considerable. It is in this sense that speech and language development at this stage represents a critical point. Once again we see that the mother-child emotional relationship has a paramount role. The mother, who at first has helped the infant in his complete dependence, has also later helped him to achieve separation from her. And she now helps him both to separate himself from the outside world and to communicate with it. Without his mother, the child is like an alien in a world familiar to all but himself. Everything appears to him as The Unknown.

This period is one of intense curiosity and drive to explore. The child shows curiosity toward his own body. Earlier, he has discovered it in parts. He now becomes aware of its total configuration, its oneness. In exploring himself he gets acquainted with smooth surfaces and orifices: mouth first, nose, ears, genital and urinary orifices. He discovers that pleasurable feelings are experienced in the handling of some areas, such as the genital area.

For instance, a little girl of twenty-one months discovers her genitalia while being bathed. She seeks to repeat the experience. If her mother puts a taboo on this activity, she gains a sense of the forbidden, of something wrong, displeasing to her mother. A conflict, at this point limited to the bathing situation, arises. It does not remain confined to bathing, and the child becomes apprehensive of incurring her mother's disapproval about the forbidden in other areas as well. The case of this twenty-one month old is from an actual observation, and the spread of a sense of taboo and aroused conflict was followed over a period of years.

The natural drive for exploration and acquaintance with self is again a critical point. The mother may accept it as a natural manifestation, or she may, because of her own attitude toward sex, interfere systematically with the child's every gesture and cause him to experience a strong sense of guilt. Such a mother is quick to describe the child's normal activity as masturbation, with all the connotations of dread and evil the word arouses in her mind.

The period of intense curiosity we are describing complicates life somewhat for the mother, who has to be watchful of the child, now "going into everything." To the child any investigation is possible and pleasurable, and even as anxiety precedes and accompanies each new venture, he has no sense of the physical danger attached to some of his activities. This dual attitude is related to a diffuse apprehension about the unknown, not the objective awareness of potential danger.

The curiosity is expressed not only in the motor sphere but also in language. At this time "Why" is a magic word. It is sure to bring an answer, even when the child is not waiting for an answer. At any rate, it is sure to bring the mother's attention to oneself. In general this phase is rapidly outlived. Some parents feel compelled to give an answer to each "Why," enlarging on the "Because . . . If . . . and How." But at this stage the child does not demand such elaborations.

One other word permeated with magic is "No." The child feels weak and inferior to everyone and everything in his environment. The word "Yes," difficult to articulate, has also little meaning. "Yes" carries too a notion of compliance, but "No" represents an assertion of self. With "Yes" nothing happens, but "No" brings repercussions and musters general attention. Negativism, which has been frequently reported as beginning toward the latter part of the 1 to 3 period, is connected with the sense of power attached to this magic "No."

The aggression and destructiveness of the child during this phase, which are part of self-assertion, self-realization, and separation from and communication with the outside world, are normal phases in the emotional development. An understanding of this fact goes a long way toward allowing its normal unfolding. Once again, maternal attitudes are instrumental in giving healthful or unhealthful directions.

Because the mother is not always favoring but also discouraging the child's impulses, he comes to have toward his mother an ambivalence of feelings which is quite marked toward the end of this period. This is the time when a child one moment hits his mother and the next hugs her with warmth and intensity. The ambivalence of feelings continues during the next period and will be further discussed. Toward the end of the third year evidence of anxiety as a normal manifestation is noted, and, like the ambivalence just referred to, becomes further intensified.

It can easily be seen that during the second span of time considered (1 to 3 years), foundations for emotional health or the contrary are solidly laid out. While the personality of a young child is marked by great flexibility and is subject to variations in response to internal as well as external stimuli, the core of his personality is already being stamped at this time. Feelings then are devoid of shadings, but they are intense. They are of the all-or-none order. And it is common observation that in later years patients are able under certain conditions (psychoanalysis, psychotherapy) to recover early experiences and relive them with the full intensity that marked them in the original life situation. This reliving is indeed part of the therapeutic process.

Three to Six Years. The trends which have emerged toward the end of the period 1 to 3 years further develop. The line of demarcation which stands at three years is entirely arbitrary, as we know. New facets of behavior appear, however, most conspicuous of which is the acquaintance with individuals outside of the family. Frequently, the child attends nursery school. But even if this experience is not available, the child is usually in contact with other children, in other homes, in the park, etc. And often in the last year of this age range, the child attends kindergarten. His social world broadens.

His drive and ability to communicate improves continually, and refinements in the expression of this drive are apparent. The need for sleep is lessening, and play occupies a good deal of waking time.

Many theories regarding the child's play, its meaning and its purpose have been advanced. Stanley Hall[16] stresses in the child's play the projection of the *past* and recapitulation of the stages of development belonging to earlier primitive life of man, as well as animals (crawling on all fours, hunting, climbing, etc.). The same external manifestations are seen by him in the child's play, although the primary purpose is no longer in evidence.

On the contrary, Karl Groos[17] looks upon play in the child as a kind of preparatory training and a projection of the *future* in play activities. Children, kittens, and puppies behave in the same way in this regard, according to Groos, who notes their ready-made powers at birth and their need for development. "Every play impulse is the dawn of a distinctive reality."

For Freud and the psychoanalytic school, symbolic expression of infantile erotic impulses (child opening and closing a box, fitting container and contained, fitting things into a box) are central, and indeed, the methods of child analysis are based on the observation of symbols and playing out of these symbols. The pleasure-principle which dominates a young child's life and the desire for gratification of his instinctual impulses are embodied in considerations of the child's play. The stress here is on the *present*.

A last group of students of child behavior view the function of play as sheer motor expression. Earlier students of child behavior were concerned almost entirely with this aspect.

As is often the case in matters of understanding of the child's behavior, all these theories help in an understanding of the meaning and function of the child's play. As a result of a ten-year observation study of nursery school children, it can be said that the child's play, although appearing simple enough is very complex in its expression and function.[18] There is in it a sheer pleasure of using muscles, of handling moving objects in the environment. There is the pleasurable and frustrating experience of attempts at power and mastery of the environment. There is a direct imitative reproduction of daily overt activities of self and of adults in the environment (sleeping and eating times, going through school or home activities, etc.). Echoing of adults in words and actions, not always with faithful accuracy, can be recorded. Says four-year-old Peter, "Day before yesterday will be Lincoln's birthday—George Washington was the father of our country and President Roosevelt has infansis surpralsis." There are continually interwoven in the direct overt expression, as given above, symbolic expressions which throw a light on the child's relationships to members of his family (father, mother, siblings) and others as no other medium could. The child has already learned to repress in his daily behavior impulses (erotic, aggressive, hostile) which, he has sensed, are disapproved. In his non-directed play he is constantly expressing these impulses through the means of fantasy and reality expressions, regressed behavior (being the baby, thumb sucking, drinking from nursing bottle, etc.) and behavior generally censored. Even this brief description of the function of the young child's play is sufficient to show the importance of giving the young child some free play-time.

He must have a chance to work out, in fantasy, impulses which are socially not permitted. The frequently hurled "I kill you dead!" or "The daddy's dead," are projections of wishes that may bring admonishment from his parents. They have failed to see that he has no actual desire physically to "kill" someone close to him, even as the fantasy is so vividly expressed or acted out. Removal, rather than physical annihilation, can well take care of the killing wish, even with all gory details attending.

From the age of three on, a child of normal intelligence who is not emotionally disturbed is well aware of the "make-believe" quality of his fantasies. Even as he indulges in the most fantastic projections, he retains emotional contact with his actual environment (reality), and weaves the reality in and out of the fantasy. This was shown in a study where children in free play sessions were approached by an observer who they felt was sympathetic to the fantasies and to whom they could reveal the "pretend" character of the play.[19]

This aspect of the fantasy-reality awareness is again a critical point in the long-term development of the child. The awareness is an index of normal functioning of the ego. In some severe illnesses (schizophrenia) this ego function has failed, and the failure can usually be traced to its beginnings in the period under consideration (in Freudian terminology, pre-genital). This is reported variously as the patient having been as a child "withdrawn . . . daydreaming . . . lost in his own world."

This period of reality testing and acting out of fantasy is one which often causes uneasiness in the parents. Some adults are prone to see in some fantasies evidence of "lying" and project difficulties to come (lying, cheating, and other personality traits) which may greatly trouble them. An acceptance of the child's fantasy as "pretend" and play, which he

128

does not have publicly to recognize with every theme, makes it easy for the child to go through the reality testing and the working out of repressed impulses. To the contrary, the parents' insistence on verification of the "truth" shakes the child's security with his parents, who, he feels, lack understanding and sympathy.

The child's feeling of omnipotence, already present earlier, takes on different forms now. Because he feels weak, inferior to adults, and threatened with new situations which arise continually, he puts forth reiterated assertions of powers invested in his father (and secondarily his mother) as well as in himself. Such assertions are expressions of the same drive for power. With this power he challenges the world, but parental power also represents a threat to him. This investing power in the paternal figure is a facet of identification with the father.

To illustrate: at meal time in the nursery school referred to previously, three boys and a girl (all approximately five) are very articulate about the power they invest in their father. From notes taken on the spot we read: *John:* "I got a big 'normous daddy" (at this point a comment is made by the teacher helping one of the other children who is dawdling and has not touched his meal). *Tom* has a timely suggestion about helping the dawdler. Says *Tom,* "My father could help. He can spank me. . . . Giants can kill people." *Joan* adds supporting evidence of her own, "My daddy is biggest of all. My daddy is a giant. . . . He's as big as the room. . . . He'd bump his head if he went in this room." When asked what she means by being a giant, she reveals the ambivalence of feelings which is so characteristic of this period. She bursts out, "They are bad people, excepting my daddy really doesn't bite, you see. . . . I'm just pretending he's a giant because he's so big." The third boy, *Bill,* is not going to be left out in this display of inner feelings. "My daddy is so big, big, big, big and tall. He would hit the ceiling with his head and then it would all bleed. It would bleed all over his hair, that's what." When a little girl from another table introjects that she also has a "big, big daddy," the competition does not stifle *Bill:* "Mine's taller. When he grows up he'll be bigger still."

These quotations illuminate the fantasies of the power projected into the father, the hostility toward the father, and the

129

fear of retaliation from the father, all of which are ever present in that age group and clearly audible and visible to anyone who has no inner need to block them.

The child does not only invest power in the parents, and particularly the father, but he has the need to assert himself with declarations of his own power. Three boys in the 4-5 age group are outshouting one another, when one of them (actually the smallest of the three) hits a second. "I'm the strongest man in the world. . . . Don't you hit him or I'll sock you." The boy thus addressed is not cowed. "I AM the strongest man in the world. I'll throw him away." This is a challenge to the first boy, who has his answer ready. "Popeye is the strongest man. He's the best man and he never dies." The first boy is still not impressed and reiterates, "No, I'M the best man. I AM the strongest."

Going out of the family circle has meant an extension and projection of family relationships into the new social group. However sketchy and embryonic, this is a first social test. In a group children begin to talk a great deal about "friends." What they express here is not a continuum of feelings between oneself and one or more of one's peers. They have become aware of the give and take of feelings as a necessity to be part of a group. Repeatedly they inquire whether this or that child is their friend.

A great deal of talk about this topic is heard in any nursery school group, as seen by the following quotations from five-year-olds. *John* kisses *Ellen* and asks, "Are you my friend?" Other children nearby repeat the question. Says *Ellen*, "Tomorrow I'll be friends with you. Today I'm friends with Peter." *John* consoles himself by answering, "Joy is my friend today." Now *Ellen* is a little uneasy and asks him, "Are you my friend?" *John* is going to make her pay the price of rejection. He says bluntly, "Joy is my friend; I'll be your friend tomorrow . . . I think." *Ellen* asserts her possessiveness, "If you are Joy's friend you can't be mine, not even tomorrow you can't be mine." The sensitive situation reaches a level of finality when *John* concludes, "Joy is my friend." Possessiveness with exclusion of others is a characteristic of this period and a sign of immaturity, an immaturity which is in order at this age but is to be found lingering in some adults.

The drive toward establishing satisfactory social relationships is not a smoothly developing one. Forward and back it goes, with reversions to the egocentricity of earlier stages. A five-year-old boy has broken a small key which a girl of the same age treasured. She shouts that their friendship, short-lived as it was, cannot be continued. "I can't be friends any more. It's too much. I'm just friends with myself."

The emotional relationships which are found in the family are projected, as stated earlier, in the new social group. Teachers are projected as parent substitutes, and play companions as siblings. Conflict, if it is present, finds its expression in the emotional relations within the social group.

The period under consideration is described as the phallic or oedipal phase. It was Freud who, in his analysis of neurotic adults, came to recognize the significance in the formation of neurotic symptoms of the sexual attachment of the boy to his mother and the girl to her father. This attachment is not initiated then but has its beginnings in infantile sexuality, the manifestations of which were also brought to light by Freud. A rivalry between the boy and his father, the girl and her mother, results and is found as a normal phase of emotional development. Under varied conditions the anxiety associated with this normal phase tends to generate a conflict which is the basis of neurotic illness.

There is ample evidence of the internal struggle experienced by the emotionally healthy child during the period. In a nursery group where children, as they are wont to do, act the family drama with parent and child dolls, the boy is substituted for the father for the acting out of parental love. When asked, for instance, why the boy is in bed with the mother, his answer is clear, forceful, and leaves no doubt as to its meaning. "The daddy's dead, so that's why." A four-year-old girl with average emotional communication with her mother announced brightly to her mother, "When you die, I'll marry my daddy." This is for tomorrow, not the remote future. That the child has an awareness of the love relationship between his parents is repeatedly evidenced. A five-year-old girl in the playroom places the girl doll, whom she intermittently calls by her own name, in the parents' bed with the father doll, removes the mother doll, explaining, "She (little girl) don't

131

get anything—this time the mommy has to sleep in the girl's bed." The manner in which these situations are handled by the parents has a decisive influence on the child's future emotional balance. The extremes of parental attitudes can vary from allowing so much body contact and freedom of expression with the parent of the opposite sex that the child feels intense anxiety as an outcome. On the other hand, a stern and forbidding attitude will arouse a sense of guilt and shame about love and sex.

In a realistic way the child in his home and out of it becomes aware of sexual differences. Again, here, parents play a major role in shaping the child's present and future attitudes towards sex. The child asks many questions, if he has not already been blocked by repressive parents. Questions must be answered, but the whole problem of answering the sexual curiosity of the child is not one merely of questions and answers. The child senses what the true attitude of the parents is. To illustrate, young parents with a Victorian upbringing, and themselves inhibited to the extent that they could not allow themselves open demonstrations of affection before and toward their children, have somehow acquired the notion that it is healthy for the child to see his parents in the nude. As if it were a ritual (and so it is), both parents walk about the apartment minus clothing in the morning, prior to the start of the day's routines. The little girl has many opportunities for thus observing her parents, and the impact of this observation is just a little too much for her to absorb in the face of other—less progressive—parental attitudes. There is no compensation for her in the fact that the rest of the day, if she lifts her skirt while playing with other children, her mother, a very proper and socially inhibited young lady, reprimands her with severity. The child is confused and in conflict about the double set of moral values and standards which are presented to her.

The curiosity of the child about his own origin, about conception and the birth process, is intense. It is natural that it should be. He is to himself the most important being. In the past the general attitude was that the child could not be curious about birth and there was no need to inform him, which made the subject a total taboo. Some of this attitude lingers, despite the wealth of information that is available now to young parents. Frequently, one is told that a child did not ask any questions and did not learn about the "facts of life" until such time, generally six or seven years, as he accidentally overheard from playmates or schoolmates some item of information that put him on the track. If the child has not appeared curious by that time, granted that he is of normal intelligence, it must be that somewhere along the earlier years he has had a need to repress his curiosity.

How big and powerful the parents loom in the child's inner mind is revealed by the type of dreams experienced by children in that age period.[20] Anxiety dreams are prominent. While the parents as parents appear in benevolent roles, they are also readily identified with powerful animals which threaten the child with total destruction. Often no interpretation need be constructed. The child offers it as he recounts his dream (so it is with fantasy—recall the "giant" conversation). Dreams offer an opportunity to work out feelings which are intolerable to the child during conscious states. It is significant that parents do not appear directly in hostile, aggressive, or destructive roles.

Here is an illustration. A four-and-a-half-year-old boy who was mildly inhibited and insecure reported dreams in which "big bad bears" ate him up; and he immediately dramatized the bear as doing the destructive things that he himself, as the father was engaged in doing in the play session. The identification was clear, and was later confirmed by his spontaneous defensive statement that it wasn't the father who did all these things, but the bear. Elsewhere in his record there are numerous identifications of the father with powerful destructive animals, bears recurring most frequently. Hostility toward the father, who was estranged from his family, was also frequently expressed. There are many other examples involving the sibling relationship as well, and the conflict of rivalry which finds its expression in dreams and symbolic play, not necessarily in overt behavior.

The ambivalence of the child's feelings for his parents is a normal manifestation. The boy wants to be "him," (identification with the father) and the girl wants to be "her" (identification with the mother). But at the same time they fear the parental figures and have hostile feelings towards them. Some degree or repression of the hostile feelings is normally shown, both because the child cannot afford to lose the love of his parents by intense and active expression of hostility, and because the ethics of the group do not allow such expression.

Through this alternating between the impulse to carry out a hostile act and the inner feeling that this hostile act cannot be carried out, the child develops a sense of right and wrong; i.e., his conscience or superego is emerging. The parents have played a major role in creating the inner feeling that the hostile act should not be carried out. The child incorporates moral attitudes which directly or otherwise are transmitted by his parents (introjection). In this phase of his growth he finds "the most support" from his parents, when his relationship to them is a healthy one. He can give up the carrying out of impulses that would bring him "satisfaction" only at the costly loss of love from his parents, if he is certain of their love and is able to respond to it. Outside of these confines any amount of parental censorship and pressure creates neurotic conflict.

The child becomes acquainted with death as a reality generally during this period. He is now able to perceive death not only as absence or removal, but what it is, an actual physical and total disintegration of the individual. He may have lost a pet animal or have seen some relative or family friend disappear after a varying period of illness. This first realistic acquaintance has generated anxiety, because the child identified himself or a parent with the dead.

Although he often has projected himself as an adult, he has not so far accepted the unavoidable end. His first reaction is that it cannot happen to him. The anxiety aroused in this first encounter with death is absorbed in the course of normal growth. Gradually, he can accept death as inevitable, because of all the positive satisfactions and richness of experience he can have before this outcome (derived from a sense of satisfaction in his current life experience). For some children resolution of the anxiety is delayed, and indeed in fewer cases it does not take place. These are neurotic manifestations. The individual stays fixed at a level which he has not been able to transcend.

Social relations are extended and intensified toward the latter part of the 3 to 6 year period and brought to a peak when the child enters formal schooling. At birth the physical separation from the mother was complete, and gradually other separations, now not physical, have taken place. The emotionally healthy child has become independent to a large extent and has developed the solid inner foundation which enables him to go ahead into what is, day after day, the unknown, something he has not experienced yet. His steps into the unknown can be considered as multiple separations of greater or lesser import, nevertheless successive separations. In this striving toward independence and ego-building, emotional support from his parents, and particularly his mother, has been the needed stimulus with every step.

The years from birth to roughly six years are the formative years, and it can be said that the child's personality at the end of this period has taken shape to a degree of individuation which stamps him as himself—unlike any other. Were it possible clearly to define all the resources, defenses, and in general the individual child's ways of dealing with reality at that age level, it would also be possible to anticipate his reactions in any future situation. This does not imply that the personality is conceived of as fixed and unchangeable at this point, but rather that its modes of reaction to external and internal stimuli are definable and predictable.

Six to Thirteen Years. This period is known as the latency period. Its beginning coincides with the introduction of the child to formal schooling and ends with the onset of puberty. Again let it be reiterated that the figures are arbitrary in that they represent only an average and not individual landmarks. During this latency period sexual impulses, which had found a peak in the oedipal situation, lose some of their intensity, in so far as the parental love-object is concerned. Indeed, normally, the boy, having passed through an intensity of erotic feelings toward his mother, has now detached himself from her and developed affective interests outside of his home. An excessive attachment of the boy to his mother or the girl to her father during this period can be considered a pathological manifestation. Indeed, in some few cases this excessive attachment may persist during adolescence and later years. Even with limited overt manifestations, extensive and severe internal disorganization may be present.

Sexual impulses are not so dormant as the term "latency period" would imply. Children have not outlived interest in the other sex's bodies, and there are normally mild exhibitionistic tendencies and sex play. Some degree of inhibition of erotic impulses has taken place, but coincident and related to the inhibition, we note an interest in terms applying to sexual activities. This is the time when parents will voice the complaint that the child uses "obscene" or "dirty" words. A bright-eyed, candid-expressioned little girl of ten or twelve will bring home terms she uses not always as applied to the subject they were designed for, nevertheless, quite explicit and forceful. She is likely to be severely reprimanded for it, the mother having "forgotten" her own interest in sexual terminology at the same age.

The most important development taking place during this period is the initiation to school life. This applies not only to the acquiring of knowledge, in itself a test of a child's inner freedom to use his native abilities, but also to the intensification of social life.

The child has many interests and responsibilities and is engaged in a variety of activities in the form of schoolwork and social play. He is gregarious in a characteristic way. This is a time when the "club" idea appears—an expression of gregariousness and get-togetherness. It is not uncommon to hear a child of eight or ten announcing with a serious expression, "I made up a club today." "How many kids in your club?" "Me and my friend." The gregariousness and drive to conform, which are further intensified during adolescence, have their origin here. Sometimes the gregariousness and drive to conform lead to not-altogether-approved social activities. A very bright eight-year-old boy reports general destruction by a group of boys in an unoccupied house. He rather prides himself on his own contribution, since it was important for him to be like the children of his neighborhood. "Our club busted most of the windows and I busted the rest completely." When asked why he wanted to bust the windows, he answers

136

promptly, "The reason I do these things is to keep up with the gang."

The desire to keep up with the gang may have more disastrous effects. Two brothers, ten and twelve years, while in treatment, told of anti-social activities which involved a goodly portion of the youth of the town in which they lived. Having heard of a house from which the resident had departed for hospitalization, several boys broke into the house. This was the starting point for dusk operations in which more and more boys from ten to fourteen years participated. These children were not from the underprivileged class, and indeed came from families of prominence in their community (and the majority of them not in therapy). The "loot" which was plundered by groups of two or three at a time was hidden by the boys in their very own house, unbeknownst to their parents, over a period of months. The two brothers referred to above did not present anti-social problems of significance outside of this specific instance. To retain status in their group they had "followed the leader" and become involved in activities which aroused considerable guilt, especially as secrecy from the parents was imperative.

Ego strengthening takes place, particularly in relation to demands which are put upon the child outside of his family. Support from his parents and parent-substitutes again plays an important role here. Superego or conscience development is also strengthening. The emotionally healthy child in the early part of this 6 to 13 period clearly shows an awareness of "right and wrong" preception and is able to repress impulses which heretofore have been uncontrolled. Parents are often concerned about behavior which they place under the category of stealing and lying. How completely unaware of the "mine and thine" concept a three- or four-year-old can be is reflected in the following illustration. An emotionally healthy girl of four addresses a nursery school teacher, "I'm going to tell Miss E. (head teacher) a secret. You mustn't look in my pad. I'm going to take something home. It's a pencil." The same child at six has developed a simple code of ethics which enables her to recognize what belongs to her and what does not. She is well able to accept the prohibitions attached.

While play continues to have an important role in development, school occupies the major portion of the child's waking hours. This is the age when learning difficulties make their appearance. A transitory block is not unusual and is only a reflection of the child's anxiety before a new situation. There are, however, a number of children who manifest more severe disturbances in the sphere of learning. The block here is neurotically determined and can be so severe as to cripple the total scholastic performance; its repercussions on social and emotional adjustment can be immeasurable.

During this period boys show little interest in girls. Even if a young boy echoing his older brother occasionally refers to his "girl friend," the reference is in no way reflecting the type of relationship that an adolescent expresses when he uses the same words. Boys have their interests, girls their own, and there is practically no crossing line. The boys are apt to voice contempt for the girls—"sissies" and "fuzzies" that they are (the occasional tomboy, provided she is not one's sister, rates a little more consideration). The girls return the compliment when they call the boys "drips," "boring," "crummy," and other sharp expressions currently in favor.

Thirteen to Eighteen Years. While changes have taken place during the 6 to 13 year period, especially with regard to the extension of social life and the taking on of responsibilities (school), the changes are not spectacular. The following period, 13 to 18, which has come recently to the absorbed attention of psychologists, is known for its more spectacular facets. Adolescence has become the number one interest of many sociologists, psychologists, and, to a degree, psychiatrists. The increase in juvenile delinquency and neurotic and psychotic illness during adolescence have helped build a distorted picture of the normal adolescent personality and the social and sexual problems it encounters.

Adolescence is often discussed as if it were an entirely new entity in a child's life unrelated to its foundations, the early years. It is actually a progression in the total development with specific phenomena, psychological and physical, taking place. Endocrine glands and sexual organs take on a spurt of activity which is reflected in the body appearance and functions; sexual impulses reach a degree of intensity which in itself calls for behavior changes.

Onset of puberty in our climate takes place between eleven and fourteen. Wide enough though it be, this range does not include the more exceptional instances of girls menstruating at nine or ten, or fifteen or sixteen. Physical changes attending the onset of puberty have, from the point of view of external appearance, greater repercussions on the girl than on the boy.

With the girl the enlargement of the breasts is the first to appear. It is a matter of no little anxiety to the average girl of twelve or thirteen to see that the other girls in her group have developed breasts and that she still maintains the flat chest of earlier years. Group living (school life, mostly) gives numerous opportunities for comparison which the individual girl must cope with. If she is insecure, this threat to development into womanhood can be disturbing. Every mother of an adolescent girl is familiar with the demand to purchase a bra long before there is any need for it, this after a repeated inquisitiveness into the promise of bulging lines. The reverse is also, though less frequently, true: a girl rejects evidence of approaching womanhood to the point where her mother finds it "indecent" that she go about without the required support. The drive to conform also plays a part, since the girl is often the butt of derisive comments when she doesn't show puberty signs at the same time as the majority of her group. Pubic hair and axillary hair put in their appearance after breast development, but being less conspicuous, delay in their appearance is less consequential.

For the boy pubic hair is the first to appear, and its configuration is on a different pattern than pubic hair in the girl, with midline hair a conspicuous feature. The genital organs become enlarged, and this is often a matter of concern for the adolescent boy, again because of group living and its opportunities for comparison. The early rivalry with the father may be reactivated. Axillary hair is last to appear and completes the cycle of secondary puberty changes.

Since the rate of development is not uniform, fixed, and strictly predictable, there is no one pattern of development applicable to all. This makes for the possibility of additional anxious reactions. Owing to increased glandular activity secretory functions of the skin are altered to the extent that skin eruptions (acne of adolescence) very frequently appear. Again a possible source of anxiety, especially at a time when social life takes a specific turn toward boy-girl relationships.

Body growth during this period also varies greatly from one individual to another. The fourteen-year-old boy who has grown very little during the preceding years is very often concerned and cannot be reassured that he may, during the next year or two, grow inches. The reverse is also true. A boy may find himself nearly six feet tall at fourteen or fifteen, and, computing how tall at that rate he is going to be when he's eighteen, becomes justifiably alarmed about this phenomenon. Dramatic situations may even develop as seen in the following incident. A thirteen-year-old boy, who was just under six feet, was once walking along a parkway in well-worn dungarees. He was stopped by state troopers who would not believe that he was only thirteen. Brought to the police station, he was kept there until his parents arrived to retrieve him. While this is an exceptional instance, it sharpens the discrepancy between physical appearance and level of personality attained with its ensuing consequences. Little reassurance can be given to the adolescent about statistics on development variations. As far as he is concerned it is, in the meantime, his own personal drama.

Size and appearance play a great role in social adjustment and emotional inner comfort. An adolescent who is somewhat oversized gives the impression of being more adult than he actually is and is expected to function at a level of emotional maturation which he has not reached. Conversely, the family and people outside of the family—school and friends, tend to infantilize the adolescent who is undersize and appears younger than his years. At the same time they reject him for the infantilization and its nonconforming, calling him "sissy, fruit, queer," and other disparaging epithets. The child who is secure with himself and his parents can more easily confront discrepancies and conflicts aroused. When the parents of an adolescent are aware that emotional maturation doesn't present one fixed immutable pattern, and they allow for individual variations, they are giving support to their son or daughter. Parents often have a rigid image in mind of what their youngster's behavior should be, mostly by comparing him with others. Whether or not they consciously formulate the wish that their child conform to the image is irrelevant. A child can feel guilty about failing his parents, even if his parents have not, in words, indicated their expectations.

In the boy alterations of the voice take place during the early part of the adolescent period. This, like other changes, can be a source of considerable uneasiness for the adolescent. Again, since there is no fixed chronological level for these alterations, parents do not help matters when they point to other boys exhibiting different patterns. The writer has known of not a few cases of boys straining so hard to lower the pitch of their voice in an effort to sound more virile, that they caused physical damage to their vocal cords. The drive to assert one's virility by forcing one's voice into a lower range than is physically possible is usually associated with a sense of physical inferiority and a desire to assert one's maleness.

Adolescence is the age of mood swings. The adolescent one day is "on top of the world" and harbors vast projects about himself, his life, and even reconstruction of the world. The next day he may be depressed and have a sense of futility and worthlessness which just as rapidly vanishes as the first mood did. This is the age (sometimes never to recur) of social and political ideals which are born of dissatisfaction in currently existing conditions. It is healthy that the adolescent should feel he can contribute to making a happier world, an ideal the previous generations have failed to achieve, so he feels. His wild conceptions are not tempered with the moderation that may come from long experience. His dissatisfaction with the world is to a degree an extension of his drive for separation from his parents.

He achieves complete emancipation in passing through stages of ambivalent feelings towards his parents. Even when his relationship to them has been healthy, he passes through a stage of alternately accepting and rejecting them. He accepts them for the emotional comfort they have given him and rejects them for the old-fashioned, rigid image they present to him, even as he may simultaneously realize their efforts to move with the younger generation.

The relationship between the adolescent and his parents is threatened by misunderstandings and impairment in communication. The adolescent feels that his parents cannot understand him, and parents are at a loss to understand the, to them, bewildering patterns of behavior, some of which they would recognize as part of their own earlier personality had they not rejected them.

Total emancipation of the adolescent can be slowed down through conflicts of his own. But it is also interfered with by parents who want him to remain a child. Needless to say, this represents for the youngster an additional block and source of conflict to work through. Seen in its over-all movement, the striving toward complete independence is not an evenly progressing course but again goes forward and back with oscillations of progression and regression which are sometimes disturbing to parents.

Probably the two most meaningful aspects of emotional development during adolescence are the intensification of sexual urges and the emancipation from parental control and influence. A corollary of the latter is the development of self-sufficiency and preparation for one's life work.

With the intensification of sexual urges many problems are likely to arise, both for the adolescent himself as well as in terms of the parent-child relationship. Tensions arise out of internal experiences which are new or intensified. Wet dreams, erections, sexual excitement can be disturbing to the adolescent boy. Similarly, the girl may have considerable guilt feeling owing to sexual responses she experiences. Earlier childhood conflicts, if unresolved, are likely to exacerbate these problems. There may be great difficulty for a boy to achieve a satisfactory love relationship with a girl to whom he is attracted, when there is resurgence of his earlier erotic attachment to his mother, conversely the girl with the father.

Our culture imposes inhibitions on sex impulses. On the other hand, if unsatisfied or nonredirected, sexual urges can create intolerable tension. This is likely to manifest itself in many spheres of behavior. To some extent the problem is today resolved by marriages earlier than was ever known in the recent past. Married students in medical and law school, etc., and even in undergraduate colleges, are a twentieth-century phenomenon, a revival of centuries past—with a difference: free will and the self-determination of the parties involved. Early marriages bring in their wake issues of another nature, non-readiness for parenthood and divorce being among the most conspicuous.

All degrees of sexual freedom are encountered in the boy-girl relationship. At the extreme, the consequences are far reaching and destructive, especially for the girls. The magnitude of this problem cannot be ascertained, since statistics on high school and college girls' pregnancies are not available. We get a glimpse into it through a knowledge of isolated instances. For instance, in a recent year when an upstate New York high school graduated seventy girl students, eleven of these girls were pregnant. There were five Catholic girls. The remainder were of Presbyterian or other Protestant denominations. In the case of four of the five Catholic girls, marriage with the child's father took place under somewhat forced conditions. The fifth one had an abortion. The birth of a child under such conditions is of double-edged import. Rejected by the natural mother, such a child usually finds its way into an adoptive home. This does not necessarily mean additional trauma but additional complexities to be sure, since motivation for adoption has many facets not necessarily related to the future happiness and emotional adjustment of the adopted child.

The healthy adolescent seeks the company of the opposite sex and can give and accept love and affection. Going steady is of this period. Going steady may not mean marriage is inevitable, though parents are sometimes troubled in contemplating the inevitability, when they strongly disapprove of their child's choice, unaware as they are that what appears a life-long interest may not lead to marriage vows. Parents are often at a loss to communicate to their children what they consider their wisdom about adolescent sexual problems. On the other hand, adolescents are seldom able freely to discuss these vital matters with their parents. Disconcerted parents may hover between excessive permissiveness and Victorian domination-possessiveness, an inconsistency likely to arouse guilt, anxiety, and hostility whichever extreme is shown. Moderation and common sense, uncommon enough, are the key to healthy parental attitudes.

The child who has from birth enjoyed security from the emotional support of his parents, who has thus been able to develop a strong ego, who can cope with frustration, will go through adolescence as one other phase of development. Granted, additional tensions are to be met, but the emotionally healthy adolescent will accept the hardships and the particular aches of that age together with the satisfaction and anticipations it also carries, because of the healthy inner core of his personality.

Part Four

THE EMOTIONALLY
DISTURBED CHILD

ANXIETY, NORMAL AND ABNORMAL

Hypothesis. Let us imagine for a moment a man who is living under the following conditions. His whole system of perceptions is intact; his intelligence is normal. This then is his behavior, when he is subjected to a variety of stimuli.

Stones are hurled at him; he sees the aggressor approaching with his weapons, the stones, yet he has not even winced when they were flying through the air. He does not stir. He is walking, and suddenly he finds himself on the edge of a precipice, the depth of which he is well able to fathom. Yet he does not alter his course, as if unaware of the danger. He is starved. An abundant supply of foods is within his reach, yet he remains inert. He is freezing and does not seek shelter, nor does he look about for something to be used as a body covering. He has had a happy relationship with his wife, but at this point another man has succeeded in wrenching her from him. This was after months of scheming on the part of the intruder, which our man has witnessed without apparent distress. Again he has failed to respond. Similarly, he is indifferent to the fate of his children. His mother, who has been affectionate and thoughtful of him through the years, has suddenly turned her back on him. He does not respond and seemingly is totally indifferent to this abandonment, as well as to the fate of his old mother going out into the unknown. What this man lives, if he lives at all, is a vegetative life. He does not perceive threats to the integrity of his physical and emotional self. Actually, as described here, he has no self and no integrity to defend. He neither flees from danger, copes with it, nor sets defenses against it.

The hypothesis is gratuitous. Such a man does not exist and cannot exist. Born as a human being, he could not have reached manhood, because he is not able to generate anxiety in situations which mean destruction of self. As an infant, his instinctual urges being satisfied by an alert mother, aware of his needs and on whom he depended, he would have survived. Past that stage, he had no choice. Anxiety is a psychobiological necessity. Many studies support this conception, among which the work of Goldstein can be cited.[1]

Normal Anxiety. Anxiety is a psychobiological necessity for the individual as well as for the species. Neurotic anxiety has been widely studied, but "normal" psychobiological anxiety very little, except by scientists, biologists mostly, with particular reference to animals. Cannon stands out for the research he has done on responses to danger with attending body changes: flight and fight being the two prototype responses to danger he observed in the animal.[2] Complete inhibition (paralysis and helplessness) must also be included. These responses are set in motion by and remain under the control of the autonomic nervous system. The stimulus is the anxiety generated through the perception of danger.

Cannon has extended his observations to man's emotional responses to danger. According to him, physical changes follow the arousing of anger and fear, changes that prepare man to attack or run. They are the body responses developed by man's ancestors in their early struggle for existence. Breathing deepens, the heart rate increases, arterial pressure rises, and blood rushes to the heart, the central nervous system, and the muscles. Adrenalin is secreted which, through the sympathetic nervous system, calls forth glycogen from the liver, supplying the blood with the sugar needed for energy. The body is thus readied for the instant vigorous action demanded by rage or fear.

This is the picture drawn by Cannon for reaction to massive danger in primitive man. The picture has not altered, as many wartime observations easily prove. Modern man does not encounter such dramatic danger situations in his every-day life, but danger stimuli are ever present in subtle and complex forms.

We have seen that in the infant the first anxiety-generating situation is birth. The disruption of the physical and chemical balance attained, which characterized its intra-uterine life, has given rise to the very dramatic picture. Satisfaction of the infant's instinctual urges means survival. Failure to satisfy these instinctual urges is anxiety-generating. The infant's anxiety is diffuse, undifferentiated, but intense. The whole body is involved, with total, rapid, vigorous movements of the limbs and trunk, and expansion of the lung cavity, all a dramatic index of the intensity of the anxiety experienced. The infant's helplessness to satisfy his instinctual urges makes him entirely dependent on his mother's care and perceptive-ness to fulfill his needs. The purposefulness found in most animals (instinct) is lacking, but the reactions are similar.

It has been said that the only "fears" the infant knows at birth are the fear of falling and the fear of loud noises. They are not actually fears, as the word is now understood, but are instinctive reactions to the disruption of balance and equi-librium experienced earlier. One aspect of this balance and equilibrium is freedom from shock and auditory stimuli. At this stage anxiety is as close to the instinctual reaction found in the animal as it can be. As he grows and with ex-perience a child comes to identify the object of his anxiety, and thus "fear" appears.

Life can be considered as a succession of anxiety-generating situations with danger threats and stimuli from the unknown —situations which are mastered one after the other with vary-ing outcomes of satisfaction or frustration. In the early years this is of particular importance; and in going, however rap-idly, over the emotional development of the young child, we have seen that he is continually facing new situations, with danger of threats embodied in the "unknown" more or less constant.

With each new step of development an anxiety-generating situation appears. In going through this situation, the child gets security and reassurance from his mother. One needs only to watch the baby tottering through his first steps to become aware of the diffuse, though intense, apprehension before the new venture. There is a threat of danger in the very "unknown" quality of this new situation. By the same token it is the anxiety itself which spurs the child into action and mastery of the situation. Let us recall that it is the failure to perceive danger and to react by anxiety, which held our hypothetical man in unresponsiveness and inaction. The child is spurred on to the next stage through the anxiety generated. The role of normal anxiety in growth and maturation can be seen in the child's attempts at warding off the anxiety by successive mastery of realities. This child utilizes anxiety towards constructive ends. Observations on this aspect of anxiety considered *normal* are wanting.

For the animal the role of anxiety—at this level solely biological—has been widely investigated and recognized. Self-preservation and the preservation of the species both are made possible through the animal's capacity to mobilize his defenses against threats of destruction which are everpresent. In the child the primitive biological reaction is overlaid with many complex forces which are culturally determined. The period of complete dependence on the mother and helplessness of the infant is one during which anxiety is at first of a biological nature, as with the animal. The infant expresses his instinctual needs in very simple forms, crying and total motor agitation. His needs are generally satisfied, and frustration appears when they are not. As physical and affective contact with the outer world develop, via the mother, his needs become more complex and the opportunities for frustration and anxiety-generating situations grow in intricacy as well as in number. His mother again gives him the emotional support he needs, as he confronts the unknown. Through experience the child comes to focus the diffuse feeling of apprehension onto objects which he can identify. Thus fear appears, and anxiety is given a name.

The differentiation between anxiety and fear is too well known to need elaboration. But there is a divergence of opinions in so far as the order of appearance of the two in the course of emotional development. The predominant conception is that anxiety precedes fear and that fear is learned.

Anxiety, whether normal or abnormal, is described as a

diffuse, undifferentiated apprehension before an objectless threat. The individual has a sense of helplessness before the magnitude of the threat. This applies to normal as well as abnormal anxiety. And indeed, many are the patients in severe anxiety states who describe "a sense of impending doom . . . of impending danger . . . of impending destruction," while realizing that they have no cause for objective fears.

Freud views anxiety as originating in the birth phenomenon and in the threat of castration.[3] Neurotic symptoms appear in order to ward off the anxiety, but actually fail to accomplish their purpose. Internal danger as well as external objects are responsible for symptom formation.

For Otto Rank the goal of emotional development is individuation through separation.[4] Separation causes anxiety. The birth trauma is considered the first separation, and the symbolism of birth recurs in subsequent separations at each stage of development.

For Adler the helplessness of the young child and his inferiority feelings proceed from his biological inferiority.[5] He relates the anxiety to the feelings of inferiority and the psychological growth to dealing with feelings of inferiority.

For Horney social and psychological factors in the culture play the important part.[6] The interrelationship of hostility and anxiety, with current conflict manifestations, is emphasized. Infantile origins of conflict are not given as prominent a place as in the Freudian system.

Differences in interpretations of anxiety by various students of human behavior, a few of which have been mentioned, are more apparent than real. Definitions can easily be reinterpreted on a common basis. For instance, the birth trauma is formulated by Freud, then emphasized by Rank as a separative process. Both agree, however, on the fact of anxiety. Biologically speaking, whether or not the concept of anxiety is used, there can be no question of a dramatic disruption of the biological equilibrium of the infant as it is separated from its mother. Other analogies can be worked out, indicating that the differences are more a question of emphasis rather than total antithesis.

Abnormal Anxiety. Abnormal anxiety is more commonly known as neurotic anxiety. The difference between normal and neurotic anxiety is not only a question of the magnitude but of the nature of the anxiety and the way it manifests itself. Freud's formulations about the appearance of neurotic symptoms as a result of failure in warding off the anxiety, even as the original purpose of the system was to do so, and the arising of internal conflict have revolutionized the concept of mental illness. Symptom formation, a device of psychological economy, does not fulfill its purpose. On the contrary, it brings to the patient additional discomfort and cause for inner conflict.

Social pressures are in constant opposition to instinctual forces related to self-preservation and species continuation. Internal danger, as well as danger from the outside, are operating at a personality level which is not conscious. For self-preservation and self-realization, however, the individual is compelled to deal with the anxiety. This he does through a multiplicity of mechanisms which will be briefly examined. For purposes of convenience they are taken up separately, but this dissociation is arbitrary, since they present themselves in complex intermingling and interreaction.

Mechanisms Used in Dealing with Anxiety. In the case of both normal and neurotic anxiety, though to different degrees, *utilization* to constructive ends is present, most conspicuously in the case of normal anxiety. So it was with the baby tottering at his first steps. Every new social approach of the pre-school child can be thus interpreted. For instance, the young child is at once anxious about a new playmate or a new adult but also attracted by the experience ("adventure"). Much of this mechanism is also in evidence in the young child's play. A child, apprehensive in the mastery of reality situations, will play out this anxiety over and over in a theme of his own to feel more comfortable about it eventually. Parents are sometimes puzzled by the apparent duality of this attitude. They may ask, "How could he be afraid of heights? He doesn't miss a chance to peer down from our tenth-floor window." Indeed, it is precisely because of his anxiety and in attempting to deal with it that he seeks, again and again, exposure to the danger.

Abreaction, another mechanism used in the handling of anxiety, is in evidence in the example just given. And again, a large part of the young child's play includes the abreaction of painful affects, in particular anxiety and aggression. The acting out of gruesome stories in which the child is either devoured by or devours animals or human beings, the acting out of ghosts' murderous deeds, of kidnappers intent on destroying them, etc., all are attempts to work out painful affects which cannot be tolerated. Here anxiety relates to the destruction of the self.

Regression is another mechanism which is clearly discernible in the young child, but continues to operate at any state of development, and most conspicuously in neurotic and psychotic disease. One is familiar with the young child's reaction to the birth of a brother or sister. He may lose bladder control temporarily, he may revert to thumb sucking, and in general behave in infantile ways he has long outgrown. Normally this phase is short-lived, and the child, after enjoying the satisfaction of being a baby again, resumes behavior at his own age level. The child who was insecure in the first place and has harbored enough anxiety (whether it has been detected or not) will continue for a longer period and sometimes become fixed at this infantile level. In the latter case, regression, initiated as a safety device to deal with painful affect, fails to fulfill its end and, indeed, reinforces the neurotic conflict.

Displacement is another one of the attempts under scrutiny. Observations of young children again provide us with many illustrations of this mechanism, which in the adult is not often so clearly or directly manifested. The writer has reported observations on the play of young children as it revolved around the family drama.[7] Numerous notes on this mechanism were entered in the records: a young child who in his overt behavior cannot afford to be hostile toward his baby brother or sister, in the playroom clearly expresses his hostility toward the baby. Although the baby is presented as A Baby, slips of the tongue or transitory appropriate naming reveal that A Baby is actually his baby brother or sister. Even if he did not reveal a name, the total context of his play would be enough to show that the original affect has been displaced. The following illustration is given of a little boy, four years old, who was travelling on an ocean liner with his parents. He was disciplined by means of threats, one being that he would be taken away by the "man with the robe" (a monk travelling on the ship). The boy played the following game. On deck he would kneel down by the hawse pipe, wide-eyed with terror, looking at the hole leading straight down to the sea. Shaking his finger threateningly as if at some imaginary person, he would say, "If you are naughty the man with the robe will throw you down there." Stepping back, he would assume a meek voice and answer, "I won't do it again, Mommy, I promise." The double role went on for some time in a game which was eventually to relieve some of the painful anxiety.

Projection, also one of the simple mechanisms in the young child, can be noted with ease. Who has not heard tales of this type? A boy full of hostility, which he dares not and cannot express in the face of strict parents, gets into numerous difficulties at school, because of his aggressive behavior. He comes home with tales of a "bad boy" (not himself, of course) who is the terror of the class. He gives this boy a name (not his own), but in the telling often comes very close to a description of himself. It is himself projected into another child, who, more often than not, is mild and non-aggressive. Similarly, a very shy, anxious child can present with relish the hostile deeds of an actual or fantasied playmate whom he is investing with the hostile, destructive, aggressive feelings that he himself feels inwardly and represses. Feelings intolerable to one are projected into another, serving the purpose of allaying one's own anxiety about such feelings.

Introjection is a mechanism similar to projection, but the direction is reversed. The concept of introjection was introduced by Freud. The child absorbs and incorporates parental attitudes and ethics, making them his own. Thus are moral attitudes developed in the young child. In the words of Freud,

This objective anxiety is the forerunner of the later moral anxiety; so long as the former is dominant one need not speak of superego or of conscience. It is only later that the secondary situation arises, which we are far too ready to regard as the normal state of affairs; the external restrictions are *introjected*, so that the superego takes the place of the parental function, and thence forward observes, guides and threatens the ego in just the same way as the parents acted to the child before.[8]

Identification can be considered next. It is also familiar to the student of child psychology. The identification process is a stage in the emotional development of the child, and one of its functions is to relieve the anxiety which proceeds from the weakness and helplessness of the child, as has been discussed earlier. There is more than a question of imitation in the stance, gait, and mannerisms of a puny twelve-year-old boy who manages to evoke the approach of his six-foot, physically impressive father. There is more to it than the aping of a physical appearance. He identifies with him. He is his father. His own weaknesses, his apprehensions recede in a background harmless to him when he "is" his father.

Repression is the basic mechanism used in dealing with anxiety, and all those enumerated above can be considered more apparent and fairly directly observable manifestations of the phenomenon of repression. As is well known, the concept of repression at a level lower than the conscious mind was formulated by Freud. Observations of patients with conversion hysteria led him to the discovery of the unconscious and of repressive mechanisms which are basic in neurotic conflicts.[9] The child is born with the capacity for anxiety—biological—which assures self-preservation. However, anxiety can be of such magnitude as to render the individual helpless. Defenses must be set for his protection.

Freud established three areas of the mind, the unconscious or id, the preconscious, and the conscious. Out of the id in the course of growth the ego emerges. The separation of the ego from one part of the id is achieved "by means of repression-resistances. But the barrier of repression does not extend into the id; so that the repressed material merges into the rest of the id."[10] The ego as the sense organ of the whole mental apparatus is intermediary between the outside world and the id. Freud regards "the ego as that part of the id which has been modified by its proximity to the external world and the influence that the latter has had on it, and which serves the purpose of receiving stimuli and protecting the organism from them, like the cortical layer with which a particle of living substance surrounds itself."[11] It then fulfills a double function, as controlling device for instinctual satisfaction (pleasure-principle of the id) and as connecting link with the external world. Control of motility and reality-testing entail a slowing down of the drive for fulfillment, with attending repression. The repressed material is stored in the id and remains accessible to certain methods of investigation (free association, psychoanalytic therapy). Freud came to the knowledge of repression through his investigation of dream material, slips of the tongue (or the pen), and other phenomena which reveal the unconscious.

The superego is generally, though loosely, equated with the conscience. It is that part of the human mind which is concerned with moral values, these values having been incorporated from parental images. Freud visualizes the ego as hemmed in between the id pressing for pleasure or satisfaction and the superego demanding the acceptance of moral values. Actually, Freud refers to "three harsh masters," namely the external world, the superego, and the id. "When the ego is forced to acknowledge its weakness, it breaks out into anxiety; reality anxiety in face of the external world, normal anxiety in the face of the superego, and neurotic anxiety in face of the strength of the passions of the id."[12] At this early stage of his concept, a hiatus was left between the birth anxiety and the anxiety later arising out of the ego function (neurotic anxiety).

Birth is considered by Freud as the first loss—loss of the mother. For him,

> every stage of development has its own particular conditions for anxiety; that is to say a danger situation appropriate to it. The danger of mental helplessness corresponds

156

to the stage of early immaturity of the ego; the danger of loss of object or of love corresponds to the dependence of the early years of childhood; the danger of castration to the phallic phase; and finally, fear of the super-ego, which occupies a special position, to the period of latency.[13]

For Freud, anxiety in a danger situation is two-fold: preparedness for defense against danger, and the anxiety itself which tends to interfere with appropriate action. The interference is caused by the residue of past experiences of which the birth trauma is the prototype. The biological usefulness of the original anxiety in stimulating at birth cardio-vascular and respiratory functions is no longer needed, but memories of accompanying anxiety are stored up in the unconscious, forming the residue here referred to (memory traces).

The ego has multiple functions. One of them stressed by Freud is to give the danger signal which sets repression processes into action. Repression plays a dual role, on the one hand in sparing the individual anxiety, and on the other, in the storing up of painful experiences by which it increases the chances for anxiety in subsequent situations.

Sublimation. According to Freud, instinctual urges are deviated from their goal, desexualized, to find outlets other than their original aims—outlets more acceptable to the ego. To some extent the process is the reverse of that of repression. Whatever school of thought, anxiety both as a dynamic and a destructive force in the emotional development of the individual must be reckoned with.

Conflict between instinctual impulses and social demands (the first social demands are parental demands) is successively resolved in the course of normal emotional maturation. The emotionally healthy child is able to pass into successive stages of development—though not as graphically as this wording would imply. Anxiety has been the leavening which spurred him on to each successive stage. He has been able to deal with it in constructive ways toward his growth.

The emotionally disturbed child, on the contrary, is in a state of conflict, the origin of which may be traced (usually retrospectively) to an earlier phase of his emotional development. The story of emotional disturbances in children is a story of anxiety and how it is dealt with by the individual child, under the usual or unusual stresses of his life circumstances (among which the parents are paramount).

EMOTIONAL DISTURBANCES

EMOTIONAL DISTURBANCES OF THE FIRST YEAR

Pioneering Research in the Field of Emotional Life in Infancy: It is no longer incongruous to speak of emotional disturbances of the first year of life. Infants in the past have not been considered capable of emotional reactions. More recent observations, however, have enlightened us on the fact that the infant is, indeed, capable of intense, if primitive, emotions, and that disturbances in the mother-infant relationship are of grave consequence to the infant. Universally recognized now are the anxiety (still referred to on occasions as fear) and rage. Depression is of still more recent import. The positive emotion should not be left out, that which comes from satisfaction of instinctual urges. One glance at a baby, previously wet and hungry, who has been diapered and has just finished his bottle in his mother's arms suffices to give an awareness of the satisfaction and contentment gained.

While the time has passed when the infant was denied any emotion, we still have very little knowledge of the infant's emotional satisfactions and frustrations and their effect on later development.

As a rule, emotional disturbances of the first year are not detected contemporaneously. However, in severe emotional illnesses of later childhood years, adolescence, and adult life, such disturbances can be recognized and brought out in retrospect. We are indebted to Spitz for an understanding of severe emotional disturbances found under certain conditions during the first year of life. In a study of the effects of institutional life on infants he observed two groups, one of infants in a foundling home and one of infants in a nursery.[14] Although physically and mentally healthy upon entering, the former children developed subsequent psychiatric disorders. Later they became asocial, delinquent, feeble-minded in appearance, psychotic, or in a general way "problem children." In the home, despite impeccable physical conditions, the susceptibility for infections and illness was great. The mortality rate was high. Very few of these infants walked, talked, or ate alone at the normal time. All were incontinent at the end of two and a half years. If we look back for a moment at Ribble's work, we will understand this state of affairs.

The condition of the children in the nursery was in striking contrast. There the infants remained physically and emotionally well. Although the physical set-up of both institutions was about the same, there was one significant difference. There, care was provided by the mothers themselves, or by adequate mother-substitutes, whereas in the foundling home all care fell upon the nurses, six nurses for forty-five children. These children were deprived of emotional interchange with their mothers; their perceptual and affective world was limited by a lack of human contact.

A follow-up study of these foundling children was made by Spitz.[15] Their mental and physical development was retarded. Their resistance to disease was low. Although the original lack of mothering was later corrected, the damage could not be undone.

Depression was observed by Spitz in infants under one year of age, a reaction he described as anaclitic depression.[16] Anxiety was also present.[17] Symptoms developed during the next six months of life were apprehension, sadness, weeping, lack of contact, rejection of the environment, and withdrawal. The infant's development is retarded, with a delayed reaction to stimuli, slowness of movement, dejection, and stupor. There may be loss of appetite, a refusal to eat, and an accompanying loss of weight. The infant frequently suffers insomnia.

The common etiological factor in these cases of depression is significant. All infants had one thing in common. They had been deprived of their mother from the age of six to eight months for an almost unbroken period. All suffered the loss of the love object. Spitz considers the resultant depression as associated with the inadequacy of the ego, at this time unable to deal with the deprivation. Motility may offer an outlet, and where motility is repressed, the infant's aggressions are turned inwardly to the self.

According to Spitz, anxiety in infants shows a rapid increase from birth to one year. At birth the ego is not present and anxiety proper does not appear, that is, anxiety stemming from a conflict between ego and id. This is in accord with Freud's formulations. However, a kind of preliminary anxiety can be observed, a state of body tension leading to diffuse discharge phenomena.

From the third to the eighth month the anxiety responses become more specific. The infant shows a "fear" in the face of both physical and psychological stimuli and reacts by drastic attempts at flight. The ego development has begun. There is also a beginning memory. Unpleasant stimuli are thus thought of as "remembered" threats.

During this second period the infant has become aware of externals, of objects, but these are yet interchangeable. From eight months to a year the infant becomes aware of the mother object as mother, a person. Being a part of the child's ego, its loss is a severe narcissistic trauma. The fear of such a loss is associated with the infants' anxiety at this time. The responses now are in the nature of anxiety proper.

During the period of eight months to a year certain psychopathological syndromes related to anxiety appear. Marasmus occurs in the third month in infants separated from their mothers, and it is during the latter half of the first year that anaclitic depression occurs. These attacks of anxiety are accompanied by severe autonomic manifestations. The child may sit in a daze, without interest in anything, exhibiting the suspicious behavior often seen in severe paranoiacs.

No description could give a better index of the intensity of feeling met with in infants than the consequences of maternal deprivation as pictured by Spitz. While some of his conclusions may appear speculative, he has brought to light numerous observations which rest on solid fact. Other observers have brought additional evidence to support his thesis, such as Goldfarb,[18] Bowlby,[19] and Aubry.[20]

Observations reported thus far have been made by a psychoanalyst and a psychologist. It is of interest to note that pediatricians in recent years have also become aware of emotional disturbances which occur in the first year. For instance, it has come to be recognized that anorexia of the infant is not necessarily physically determined. Levesque[21] speaks of a "true neurotic anorexia" (my transl.), differentiating this type from two other conditions: 1) secondary anorexia, which is subordinate to another illness and terminates with that illness, 2) essential anorexia, associated with digestive disorders and vitamin deficiency usually occurring from six months to two years, in the absence of psychogenic factors.

True neurotic anorexia may be transitory, usually occurring with changes in the child's feeding. Psychologically it may be related to the parents' lack of warmth and interest or the arrival of a sibling. It is likely to terminate when the environmental factors are recognized and can be improved. However, there is also a more severe and chronic form which has its beginnings in the first week of life and takes on the pattern —now known to the reader—of food refusal, lack of interest in sucking, occasional vomiting, and concomitant signs of anxiety. This anorexia of the infant, in the experience of Levesque, usually disappears at from two to five years but can persist until adolescence or even later. While he does not go into the psychodynamics involved, he points out the relationship between the parents' neurotic personalities and the tendency of these infants to develop, at a later stage, severe personality disturbances of their own.

A more extensive and perceptive study was reported by a pediatrician and his associate, Debré and Mozziconacci.[22] These authors carefully studied the frustrations of infants' psychological needs which so often go counter to the feeding methods used. It must be recalled that in the first year, especially the first part of it, the essential contact of the infant with the outside world is through its mouth. Rigid schedules impose rigorous quantities, times, as well as behavior patterns which may or may not fit with his needs. Sight, smell, and taste, while essential to all infants in their contact with the outside world, vary from one infant to the other.

"Frustrations of psychomotor development" and "frustrations of affective needs" are also considered by these writers. Throughout, it must be remembered that the infant's satisfactions come primarily at the oral level, and that severe frustrations can occur, if recognition is not given to the infant's oral needs. The study attempts to differentiate between certain types of mothers with "disturbed maternal instincts . . . obsessional over rules of hygiene, timing, etc." (My transl.). These mothers may be rejecting or overprotective. The writers feel that "an intellectual mother can drive a child to anorexia," as over-intellectualization is often associated with "instinctual poverty." They also consider some mothers infantile, dependent on their husbands as they were on their parents, with the infant representing a rival.

Further comments are of interest, such as the predominance of anorexia among girls—the strong tie between the mother and female child, with close identification a determining factor. In their view, there is too much regimentation of feeding in our modern world, with individual variations and factors of psychomotor and affective development overlooked. They point out that anorexia is a disease of modern civilization. They find not a trace of it in medical writings before the end of the last century. First seen almost exclusively in well-to-do families where rigid patterns of infant care were early adopted, it spread with time through other classes. The rigidity brings frustrations in its wake.

We have seen that very dramatic conditions of both physical and psychological order can develop from maternal deprivation. By and large these conditions are not everyday occurrences in the practice of pediatricians or psychiatrists. The average child psychiatrist seldom encounters the dramatic effects described by Spitz, since these are observable under very special life conditions (nurseries, infant homes, etc.). Their very dramatic quality serves to enlighten and emphasize the effects of deprivation which, for the general mass, are encountered in varying degrees rather than in their totality.

Emotional disturbances of the first year are expressed biologically, which is readily understood, since ego development

163

does not begin until the latter part of the first year, as briefly discussed earlier. When the instinctual urges of the infant are not fulfilled, certain manifestations, both physical and affective, appear. They are so intermingled in their expressions, however, that it is obviously arbitrary to present them as separated. In all physical manifestations the affective element is present. Conversely, affective manifestations utilize the various physical systems. It is a question of emphasis on one element or the other rather than complete separation of the two.

The *motor function* can be stimulated or slowed down. Motor restlessness, head banging, rocking, and motor listlessness are some of the more prominent indications. Head banging and rocking deserve special attention. In taking the history of some severe emotional disturbances (early infantile autism, schizophrenia), one finds that they are seldom missing. If an infant is deprived of maternal body contact, the frustration is likely to manifest itself in intense body self-stimulation. These body movements should be differentiated from pendular motion found in congenital mental deficiency, where the picture is at various (repetitiveness without tonicity). In the case of the emotionally disturbed child, while there may be a pendular-like rhythm in head banging and rocking, the goal of body stimulation is primary. The muscular tonicity characteristic of these activities is witness to the motivation. In contrast to the motor restlessness and increased motility here described, one may find a diminution in motor activity together with degrees of apathy and affect withdrawal, the extreme of which has been decsribed by Spitz as anaclitic depression.[23] There is no difficulty in recognizing the affective quality of the decrease in motor activity.

The *gastro-intestinal system* can be a focus of expression for affective disturbances, constipation and diarrhea being some of the symptoms. At this stage, excessive thumb sucking is one of the conspicuous expressions of frustration, and in its turn can bring a variety of gastro-intestinal disturbances as a result of insufficient nutrition.

The *respiratory tract* can also be involved. *Breath-holding spells* are encountered in the early history of many children with anxiety syndromes of early childhood. We have seen that respiration is one of the incomplete and inadequate functions at birth. Body tensions resulting from lack of instinctual satisfaction can more readily appear in a lesser than a better organized system. For an all-inclusive description of the syndrome and its varied causes, one should turn to the classic description given by Kanner: "There are episodes in the course of the first four or five years in the lives of some children in which, mostly in the midst of violent crying, they suddenly stop breathing and do not resume respiration for the length of about half a minute. During this time the child frequently becomes cyanotic, especially around the lips and face."[24] Secondary signs sometimes occur, apnaeic distress with random movements of the limbs and anxious expression. The eyeballs may be turned upwards. On rare occasions associated movements are also noted, such as twitching and jerking. The movements may be restricted to the face or they may spread to the whole body. If the breath is held extensively, the child loses consciousness and falls backwards with a very rigid, or conversely, a limp and lifeless body. Should the attack be extreme, severe convulsions are likely to take place. Following the attack, the child, provided he has not lost consciousness, may either continue to cry or show total exhaustion. Kanner, analyzing the psychodynamics of these breath-holding spells as found in later years (under five), finds that "breath holding is usually one of several signals of a disturbed parent-child relationship." Needless to say, the dynamics are here studied contemporaneously to early childhood, and not infancy.

Following on the value of breath holding as a disturbance signal, Kanner further comments,

Many of the parents are found to be overprotective and oversolicitous. Many of the infants are found to be generally resistive and remonstrating especially against a tense and rigid feeding regime and prematurely enforced regulation of toilet habits. When this type of relationship persists, breath holding, which almost always ceases at or before four years of age, is replaced by temper tantrums or crying spells.[25]

Kanner reviews the multiple causes (organic as well as affective) of this syndrome. Here we are concerned with it only as a manifestation of an emotional disturbance.

Any body system can be involved in the expression of anxiety. Let us single out the *urinary tract,* not because of its greater frequency, but because several cases have come to the attention of the writer where a background of severe emotional disturbances caused urinary retention. One will be described at length under the next chronological group. These urinary disfunctions, while beginning during the first year, are usually detected later.

The eczema of infancy is also associated with early emotional disturbances, although this again is not usually so diagnosed contemporaneously. A large number of neurotic problems encountered in post-infancy years reveal in their early history the presence of eczema. Studies of psychogenic factors in asthma and eczema are now well known in so far as the older child and adult are concerned.

Usually the various somatic manifestations here briefly presented are investigated from the point of view of physical causes. During the first year of life the investigation is very seldom pursued into the realm of psychodynamics. From the second year on, approaches to early emotional disturbances of children, when they are expressed somatically, take on the following pattern: exhaustive study of possible physical causes with laboratory, dietary, physical examinations, etc., and final recourse to psychiatric treatment. Additional traumata resulting from these approaches need no elaboration. Not that an exhaustive physical study is unwarranted, but the emotional climate in which the somatic manifestations are developed should not be overlooked.

Early emotional disturbances can be present with the affective component overshadowing the physical expression. This is no guarantee that they will be recognized contemporaneously either. In collecting anamnestic data of severely disturbed children or adolescents, one may gain the impression of infancy years during which the infant has been conspicuously deprived emotionally. This comes up under various descriptions such as apathy, lack of interest in people who approached the infant, etc. It is often difficult to get a clear

166

evaluation of the severity of the emotional deprivation until one has a chance to study early photographs.

The following case is not presented as a clinical study, although material available would make the presentation possible. Material has been selected to emphasize the value of observations on the first year of life through whatever medium may be available. The observations pertain to a fifteen-year-old girl with the diagnosis of paranoid schizophrenia. She is the elder of two children, the second being a boy who was born when she was close to three years of age. The boy is free from emotional conflict. The family belongs to the upper-middle-class level. Both parents were young and this was the first pregnancy. The mother, for complex reasons which need not be elaborated upon here, wanted a boy. This was not a mere "fancy," since she found it intolerable to be in the same room with the baby (if this was a boy) of any of her friends, because of the anxiety this aroused in her. She is a perfectionist, immersed in social functions in and out of her home. The father is a professional man, perhaps more of a perfectionist than his wife. He had several compulsions, one of which was carefully to check on the daily food intake and excretory functions of his children. The mother, who was disappointed at not giving birth to a boy, was said to have entrusted the complete care of the baby to a "well-trained" registered baby nurse, relying completely upon her for the care of the infant. The nurse was very busy with the carrying out of minutely outlined schedules regarding food, sleep, physical care, etc. She mounted guard near the baby, keeping away human contacts as much as was feasible except for the father, who always had a hand in the planning. The mother, by natural lack of affinity and disinterest, did not need to be kept out; the infant was brought to her at intervals. In the initial taking of anamnestic data the fact of her rejection was clearly established. It was clear that the baby's care and training was mechanically perfect, but that "mothering" was totally absent.

The extent and intensity of this rejection, however, could not be grasped and its devastating effects evaluated until a revealing photograph was later presented to the examiner. This showed a mother who had been coaxed (by her husband) to hold her baby, then six months old. The mother sits rigidly, her trunk vertical, her lap horizontal, with arms hanging down in the hieratic manner of an Egyptian statue. Her facial appearance is difficult to describe. It is expressionless, but with a turned-away, disowning look. Words can easily be placed in her mouth. They say, "What is this object lying in my lap?" The object is a six-month-old baby girl, lying totally rigid on her stomach. The body seems precariously placed on the edge of the mother's lap, one might say as a bread board on the edge of a table. The head is slightly turned to the photographer, and the eyes are so large as to suggest wide dilation of the pupils. It is obvious that the baby is in an attitude of rigid defense against overwhelming anxiety. Perhaps no description of this girl's early life could give as vivid a picture of the mother's rejection, the intense anxiety resulting, and the hunger for love as well as distrust of love which characterized the girl's incapacity for affective relation in later life.

The patient was always friendless, and her obsessive goal was to achieve perfection. She must be at the top of her class, and she was. Perhaps she could win her mother's love this way. The patient was aware of her drive for perfection as a way of getting love from her parents, primarily her mother. On several brief occasions when she succeeded in obtaining the friendship of a classmate, she was unable to sustain the relationship and she became very rapidly distrustful of the friend. She could not accept the reality of positive feelings toward herself, because of the early deprivation from the mother.

During her adolescent years compulsive sexual promiscuity appeared with the repetitive pattern: hunger for love, seeking an object, not finding love, complete inability to give love either in its tender or sexual component (sexual frigidity), being aware of this sequence, and again being driven to repeat the cycle.

The early deprivation of maternal love set the pattern. In spite of the fact that the father in part took the maternal role, the loss could never be made up. Indeed, the patient has violently resented the dual parental role of her father which made still more difficult the normal identification and has contributed to her extreme confusion in male-female identification. It is doubtful that even with the most skillful therapeutic approach these early losses can ever be made up. It must be noted also that in the therapeutic transference (if and when this takes place) this hunger for love creates its special problems, marked by excessive dependence, distrust, and even doubt that any human being could take an interest in one, whatever the motivation may be.

We have seen from Spitz's work the extensiveness of emotional trauma in the loss of the mother. In problems of infancy this loss is initially suffered.

David Levy was the first worker to call attention to these early maternal deprivations, as he became aware of them in retrospect.[26, 27] He studied them in the context of neurotic and behavior problems of older children, but pointed to the evidence of early maternal rejection and its almost inevitable concomitant, maternal overprotection, a compensatory mechanism arising from guilt feelings. He defined *affect hunger* as "an emotional hunger for maternal love and those other feelings of protection and care implied in the mother-child relationship."[28] The reader will recall Ribble's brilliant presentation of the infant's emotional needs, and its satisfaction or non-satisfaction through the effective presence or absence of mothering.

Levy, in studying affect hunger, finds its symptoms present in children who have had more than adequate systematic physical care. The cases he cites for illustration are from his own clinical experience. They had been referred during the years of childhood, at about eight years on the average, and Levy's knowledge of their actual infancy has been only through the records of institutions, the reports of nurses and social workers, and other secondary sources. In every case, however, early maternal rejection has been obvious. The histories have the following points in common: illegitimate birth, shuffling from one institution to another, from one foster family to another, and, finally, adoption.

The complaints on referral of these cases are similar, all stemming from severe affect hunger. There is a degree of delinquent behavior, sexual delinquency, stealing, fantastic lying, and there is a marked inability to respond emotionally, to give affection. Levy points out that these symptoms are to be found not only in children who have suffered lack of mothering at birth, but also in children who received mothering for the first two years, perhaps from a foster parent in an institution, and were adopted at the end of the two years. A break at this stage may make later emotional response difficult or even impossible.

Levy, as many subsequent observers will agree, comments on the irretrievable quality of this early lack. Some children, however, do find help in later years through the love of foster parents or with supportive therapy. In the latter the primary role of the therapist is to act as a substitute parent.

The unsatisfied need for affective satisfaction is manifested in various ways which can be broken down roughly into three categories, according to Levy. In the first are "a group of activities representing responses to the primary need." These activities include play for affection, kissing, hugging, clinging, and a display of helplessness. There are pleas for love, constant crying for attention, whining. In the second category are activities which "represent various hostile acts designed to punish the one who denies love and to prevent the possibility of its withdrawal." Here we can place death wishes against the mother, sadistic fantasies, threats of violence against the mother, threats of suicide. Temper tantrums and the whole gamut of "bad" behavior fall into this category. The third group of activities "are based on the child's fear of the hostile impulses." Various fears follow hostility, fears of retaliation. The most common, of course, is the fear of death. Less obvious, but still stemming from the same cause, are feelings of deprivation and of self-pity and depression.

Levy has noted cases where even the restoration of maternal love is ineffectual in bringing back any security. He has noted also, however, children who are later able to establish satisfactory emotional relations. Many children fall between these two extremes and have serious relationship difficulties because of the early lack of maternal love. The difficulties do not end with childhood. Many adults must constantly seek in every friend a substitute mother. They make fantastic demands on friendship. When the current relationship fails, they fall into a depression and a sense of loss until another one is established. In both child and adult this emotional deficiency is characterized by excessive demands "for food, for money, for privileges." The demands cannot be satisfied, and there is a need to repeat constantly the original frustration.

Levy has observed that in each case there is a particular need for a certain aspect of maternal love. One child may seek especially the protective phase of maternal love, another may seek its giving quality.

In others it may be the mere demonstration of affection, including also genital satisfaction. These elements represent special incompleteness in the early emotional development of the patient and must be demonstrable in numerous phases of the life history.[29]

Before going on with the discussion of maternal rejection, a brief account of maternal overprotection should be given. This is but another aspect of rejection, a guilt reaction resulting in excessive compensation. Levy has described the basic features of overprotection, "excessive contact, e.g., a mother sleeping with her son, aged fourteen . . . prolongation of infantile care . . . prevention of the development of independent behavior . . . lack or excess of maternal control."[30] A child brought up under these conditions is likely to be either overaggressive and egocentric or submissive and effeminate. He will show irresponsible behavior and an inability to make and keep friends.

ANOTHER CLINICAL CASE

In certain cases of maternal rejection the conspicuous defect may not appear to be affective, although it definitely is so, the presenting complaint being in the intellectual sphere. A case of this nature came to the attention of the writer and has previously been briefly presented.[31] This child was referred for treatment at the age of seven years, eight months. Her history was one of extreme emotional deprivation. Born out of wedlock in the wealthy family of the international sophisticated set, she was left behind while her mother went alone to rejoin her lover, the child's father, whom she later married. The pregnancy had taken place during the mother's second marriage and the father's third marriage. At the date of writing the child's mother and father are in their fourth and fifth marriages respectively. The child was left in a foster home, not approved by any agency, and the mother kept in touch with her via a large series of expensive photographs (a valise full of them was presented at the time anamnesis was taken).

When the child was seven and a half months old, she was, at the mother's request, visited for the first time by the nurse who had attended the mother at delivery. To the nurse the baby seemed retarded. When the baby was nine months old, the nurse arrived unannounced with a photographer and found the patient one of several babies crowded in a room (six "beds" to a room). The child herself was "in such a very narrow box that only her head could move." There was an extensive area of baldness on the back of her head due to constant rubbing (recall infant's drive to obtain satisfaction from self-stimulation of any part of the body in the absence of mothering.) When, finally, the mother and father, now married, came to see this child shortly thereafter, they were told by the pediatrician that the child was mentally deficient and should be placed in an institution. A month later the parents left the country, entrusting the infant to the care of the obstetrical nurse. The nurse described the child's condition at the time as follows.

"She didn't sit, suck, or turn her head. She had pyelitis and bronchitis, and also her jaw muscles were underdeveloped." Unresponsive to offers of feeding, the baby had to be fed with a dropper while held in the arms. Later, a small spoon was used. At the beginning it would take hours to feed her, and following feeding, she vomited. This picture is clearly reminiscent of the children described by Spitz. It will be recalled that the children given institutional care without mothering were unable to walk, talk, or eat alone. Their development was retarded; they showed a lack of appetite or even refused to eat. At one year this baby developed an allergy to most proteins (numerous skin tests were carried out).

At the age of five she was placed in a private school kindergarten. But after one week, she was rejected, because her intelligence was evaluated as that of a moron. Her I.Q. was 60.

At the age of seven years, eight months she was referred for treatment, because of the following complaints formulated by the nurse who served as mother-substitute. She showed extreme motor restlessness and an inability to concentrate. Her school-work was very poor. She had an allergy in the form of bronchial attacks of several years' duration. The other complaints were stealing, smearing of feces, and intra-rectal manipulation, both at home and at school. The child's psychomotor development was retarded, a fact readily understood.

Under the warm care of the nurse and with the help of psychotherapy, improvement in all areas was noted. By the age of eight and a half, psychological testing showed her I.Q. to be 82. The symptoms for which she had been referred had decreased, the smearing of feces and intra-rectal manipulation having stopped completely. Her school record showed slow improvement.

One must look back to Ribble's observations on the importance of mothering in the development of the brain, which at birth is very immature. The girl just described was totally deprived of mothering during the first nine months of life and was also physically neglected. Love-deprivation and the absence of mothering, in addition to physical neglect, contributed to the picture of undeveloped intellectual function noted at the time of referral.

For the sake of brevity only a few notes from the therapeutic sessions have been lifted because of their relevancy to the early emotional deprivation and its traumatic effects. It was some time before the child responded to affection. There was an enormous preoccupation with death. Frequent references to "funeral house, grave box" made me feel even then that, although she could not describe early surroundings, the symbolism was determined by memory of her infancy life-conditions. She acted out again and again the mother-child situation, emphasizing maternal duties. "I'm the mother . . . The mothers have always to wash their babies." She was in

173

turn a possessive, loving, and scolding mother. Recalling her early experience in the confining crib of her infancy, such statements and acting out as the following are of great interest. How can these statements which frequently recurred in her play be but a recall of "body memory"? "Here is all the crib stuff because you have to be locked in because you are baby . . . because you might fall out of bed . . . same when I was a baby, I remember." (This at a time when she had assigned the role of baby to the therapist.) The mother-child relationship, with its many facets revealed at unconscious levels, was played over a period of months. In addition to the warmth she was getting from the mother-substitute, she gained security and in the therapeutic situation resolved some of her problems. This was reflected in her scholastic improvements.

Unfortunately, she left after fifteen months of therapy. The mother, incapable of giving love to this child, had come to resent the girl's attachment to the nurse as mother-substitute. At intervals and arbitrarily, she summoned the child with her nurse to her current home. She showed her to her friends, got impatient with her antisocial behavior, and sent her back with the same dispatch as she had been summoned. The child, incidentally, was and still is very beautiful.

Shortly after this the mother decided to place her in a boarding school, and over a period of years she has been in a number of boarding schools with therapy and without. Therapy, however, has never been carried out consistently and was arbitrarily interrupted by the mother at intervals for her own needs to show off her daughter, who, on first impression, was indeed attractive. Both mother and father meanwhile had divorced and remarried in the proportion earlier described. Throughout the years this girl has never had any emotional roots. She feels rejected by both parents, and her ambivalent feelings toward them is mostly intense hatred which she verbalizes freely.

This patient would have been lost sight of completely but for the fact that, while her mother was on one of her cross-continent travels, the girl became involved in a serious situation which brought her back to the attention of the writer. Then close to nineteen, and ten years after her therapeutic contact with the writer, she had been at a new boarding school for only two months, when she was threatened with expulsion because of sexual promiscuousness. As far as the school was concerned, the promiscuousness was of a homosexual nature. But it later became known that she also had picked up male strangers in the street and become sexually involved on trips to and from the school.

She was then entrusted to her guardian, a respectable, conventional man, at whose home she occasionally stayed for short vacations with his wife and children. The girl's sexual aggressiveness toward him prompted this man to seek advice. She was not seen at this time, but the picture as described was one of delinquency and sexual promiscuousness as a compulsive manifestation, a repetitive pattern which has been described in relation to another case.

For obvious reasons this case can only be sketchily presented. Nevertheless, certain facts stand out: the early deprivation which was never compensated for, affect losses which could never be regained, although intensive and long-continued therapy might have made it possible for her to develop some inner core in an integrated personality. Intensive therapy in a psychiatric hospital, which was suggested at the last contact, was probably not carried out.

We have seen that Freud considers the first appearance of anxiety in connection with birth. This anxiety is recognized by all, including Freud, as biological in nature. The appearance of neurotic anxiety, according to Freud, requires the formation of the ego. It is obvious that between the birth anxiety (biological) and the appearance of neurotic anxiety depending upon the formation of the ego, there has been a hiatus which is now rapidly being filled in, mostly by Freud's followers.

Spitz's work was pioneering in this area and in this sense also revolutionary in the revamping of the concepts of mental illness. It stimulated widespread interest in the first year of life, and a number of studies have since appeared which stress the importance, from the point of view of emotional development, of the mother-infant relationship. This new orientation was brought into focus at the International Institute of Child Psychiatry, Toronto, 1954 (in effect the second International Congress of Child Psychiatry, the First International Congress of Child Psychiatry having taken place in Paris in 1937). Probably nothing can illustrate better the progress which has been made in the understanding of childhood and adolescent (and therefore adult) mental illness than these two landmarks do.

At the First International Congress the majority of papers were concerned with "neuropsychiatric constitution and . . . conditioned reflexes . . . special methods of education for mentally retarded . . . consideration of educational approaches for children with intellectual and personality difficulties . . . studies on juvenile delinquency . . . aspects of forensic psychiatry," and, on the whole, very little of psychodynamic considerations and not a trace of interest in the first year of life.

In contrast to this picture, the International Institute of Child Psychiatry, 1954, in Toronto, was almost exclusively concerned with the psychodynamics of the earliest years ("emotional problems of children under six"), the mother-child relationship, and its disturbances. The program was divided into three parts:

I. Preventive Aspects of Child Psychiatry
II. The Relation of Physical and Emotional Factors and Problems of Hospitalization
III. Problems of Psychosis in Early Childhood

Each section was made up of two parts: clinical cases and research reports.[32] It is of interest that, while the Institute was dealing with the problems of children under six years, roughly half the papers were concerned with the first year of life—the first year in its most meaningful aspect, the mother-infant relationship. Actually, psychiatrists have little chance to observe emotional disturbances of the first year, since the child at that age is usually under the exclusive care of the pediatrician. However, in the majority of cases presented at the Institute, the psychiatrist presenting a case had been as close to the first year of life as any psychiatrist might have. One is impressed again and again with the damaging effects of a disturbed mother-infant relationship, effects manifested both somatically and emotionally.

EMOTIONAL DISTURBANCES
OF THE ONE TO THREE YEAR PERIOD

We have seen that during the first year of life anxiety, at first biological in nature, is expressed somatically or emotionally. During the 1 to 3 year period anxiety takes on new forms. As a direct manifestation—without defense—it is in a mild form very general in this age group. It may, however, be intense enough to be considered abnormal, i.e., neurotic. The normal anxiety can easily be recognized: one is familiar with the picture of a child of two or three who is approached by strangers or meeting with strange objects (large toys, animals, etc.) or entering a new situation. The general apprehensiveness is shown in the sudden rigidity (freezing) of the body attitude, widening of the pupils, and sudden blocking of speech, or rapid enunciation of words not necessarily connected or relevant. There may also be crying. This picture is well within normal limits, being, for this case, proportionate to the external stimulus (the unknown).

Its counterpart, however, as it expresses an emotional disturbance is first of all out of proportion with the stimulus. It is intense, diffuse and blocks the child's functioning; it may prevent him from eating, sleeping, moving about (or its opposite, hypermotility). It may bring the child back into a state of excessive dependence (clinging) on his mother—excessive in that he has now passed the stage of complete physical dependence and relative emotional dependence. In addition to the partial and multiple disfunction this anxiety may bring, it can also be manifested through specific organs. Perhaps the organs most involved are the excretory organs (incontinence or retention of urine—diarrhea or constipation). The mechanism of organ selection is not always clear, but in some cases, where the symptoms developed early enough after the apparent external stimulation, it can fairly easily be brought out, as will be shown.

In this age group three categories of neurotic manifestations put in their first appearance, namely, *behavior manifestations, language disturbances,* and *contact disturbances.*

The first defenses against anxiety also put in their appearance, rituals, for instance. It is normal for a young child to insist on having his favorite stuffed animal at bedtime, as a guarantee that he will fall asleep (reassurance against the mild anxiety which precedes sleep). The multiplicity and severity of rituals, however, may be such as to represent at this early stage precursors of the compulsive acts found in a severe form of neurosis, the obsessive-compulsive neurosis of the adolescent and adult.

Anxiety and Phobias. As previously indicated, *anxiety and phobias* represent probably the most common disturbance of this age group. Rather than present a number of cases with varied individual manifestations, one case has been selected for its multiplicity of symptoms. Such symptoms are found in that age group singly or concurrently in a variety of patterns.

A CLINICAL CASE

Formulation of the complaint: Elly, twenty-three months old when brought to the writer, was an only child of young parents. In her first interview the mother revealed in a few words what to her was the nature of this child's problem. Her first statement was, "She is difficult to manage." Briefly and at the onset, let it be stated that the child's difficulty was one of severe anxiety which permeated all aspects of her behavior. At no time prior to psychiatric contact had the parents recognized it as such, a fact which is common enough in psychiatric experience. For the parents, and in particular the mother, the problem was one of "management."

Going on with the narration of her problem the mother reports that the child *"screams on and off during the night and you can't stop her."* The screaming lasts for hours, and the mother comments that "people don't know how she can keep it up." Once she screamed without interruption from eleven thirty P.M. to two thirty A.M. The child, who is unusually articulate for her age, at bedtime screams, "I don't want to go to bed. . . . I don't want to sleep." She stalls with many "excuses," she must go to the toilet, she must have a drink of water, she must urinate, etc. Bedtime has become an ordeal for both mother and child.

The mother also finds her "difficult" during the day and goes on to describe *negative and contrary behavior,* asking for milk or other food and then rejecting it in a negative and see-saw pattern. *Temper tantrums* are reported, but obviously not perceived as anxiety manifestations, since the mother adds, "I spanked her so she doesn't dare." As her next statement indicates, one does not deal so easily with anxiety, slapping it out of existence: "Instead she has started *pulling her hair.*" In passing, the relationship between anxiety and self-punishment, so clearly illustrated here, is a common observation during this as well as other age periods. The younger the child, the easier it is to demonstrate the immediacy of the relationship. *The whole picture has developed progressively over a period of approximately six weeks,* according to the mother. We will see that there were disturbances of another order prior to that time.

The parents' attitude toward the child's difficult behavior has fluctuated from strict and punitive to another extreme, completely ignoring it. On occasions they have also tried to "quiet" the child, but there is no evidence that this was much more than just a gesture, nor are there indications that cuddling and affection were lavished.

The family history: The older generation, i.e., the paternal and maternal grandparents, shows definite neurotic trends. The *paternal grandfather* is said to be shy with strangers, withdrawing from social contact, although he has a few friends with whom he is capable of "warm" relationships. The statement is made that "he didn't go to the movies in years." He is mild and passive, completely dominated by his wife. He is also described as "very methodical and a little compulsive." The *paternal grandmother* is described as "the opposite of him . . . nervous," has many psychoneurotic illnesses, makes suicidal threats, using both to control her environment. She is explosive and following "very bad tempers" is contrite and asks for forgiveness. It is learned subsequently that, although the father was first reported as being an only child, a girl had been born to this grandmother prior to his birth. A "pyloric baby," she died at six weeks. When her son,

179

the patient's father, was born, the grandmother was very disappointed, for she wanted a girl. Her psychoneurotic illnesses became acutely intensified following the father's birth. When the father was four years old, the grandmother had a complete hysterectomy. She has dominated her son during his whole life, including the marriage years.

Of the *maternal grandparents* the grandmother seems to be the more stable. The grandfather is immature, sociable, subject to great mood swings, with rapid short-lived anger a prominent mood.

The *father*, an "only" child, is twenty-nine years old and was reared as a Protestant. He converted to Catholicism before marrying the patient's mother, who is a Catholic. "Of his own free will" is the mother's qualification. He must have been very much in love at the time to face the resistance of his mother. She strongly opposed his marriage, on the surface because of religious differences, but actually because of her possessive and excessive attachment to him. He is an engineer, capable of doing outstanding work, but lacks ambition. He "tends to look toward the bright side," an over-optimism which particularly defeats the mother, who is tense and pessimistic. He married at twenty-four, and despite his mother's resistance and his own passivity both of the parents assert that they found happiness in their marriage. The mother makes the reservation, "except he was not too much of a conversationalist." The paternal grandparents helped financially, and under war conditions and housing limitations the young parents lived with the paternal in-laws for a period, so the parents initially presented their short stay with the older generation. Actually, there were other and more meaningful reasons for the paternal grandmother's role in the child's early life. In addition, the father was thrown into a maternal role owing to the mother's illness, to be elaborated upon.

The *mother*, twenty-six years old, is a small, underweight (90 pounds) young woman, quiet, very tense. She is the fourth of seven children, and her middle position seems to have made her the "forgotten child" in her family. She feels that her childhood has been fairly happy, "except my mother had a lot of children." The statement about a happy childhood becomes questionable on further contact, since the mother feels that she has been "deprived of a lot of things" and has felt that way "always." She also presents a picture of intense early childhood anxieties manifested by nightmares, great fear of her father, who "had a bad temper." She found that her mother "lacked understanding" and was rough in the handling of her fears. For instance, if the child came crying to the mother's bed at night, the mother would send her back impatiently to her own room. It is clear that this young mother has had a succession of neurotic difficulties through the years. As a young child, she had been anxious and generally apprehensive. She felt great dissatisfaction during adolescent years because of her inability to enter college (her parents resisted the idea). Approximately one year before her marriage at twenty-one she developed severe "digestive trouble," which was—following her baby's birth (three years after marriage) identified as colitis. Some two years after the beginning of digestive symptoms her appendix was removed, but no improvement took place. The colitis was originally suspected, an X ray having shown significant intestinal changes a year or so after marriage. This account of physical illness must be evaluated, however, in terms of emotional conflicts, and in particular the mother's relation to her mother-in-law. She spontaneously interpolates, "I have a lot of trouble with my husband's mother, who tries to run our lives." Shortly after the baby's birth and owing to both the mother's and the baby's somatic illnesses, the family lived with the paternal grandmother. Although at the time of referral the grandmother had changed her ways and "tried to be nice," the period following the baby's birth was very traumatic to the mother. She recalls having been told by her mother-in-law that she was sorry her son had married her.

The child, her personal history: Elly was born three years after her parents' marriage, when the father was twenty-seven and the mother twenty-four. Although the pregnancy is reported as "planned and wanted," it is clear that the mother was not emotionally ready for the experience, because of her own neurotic difficulties as well as her husband's emotional immaturity and dependence on his mother. During her pregnancy, which was the normal nine months' duration, the mother was "not too well," very nervous, and had insomnia.

181

Toward the end of the pregnancy colitis became so severe that heavy doses of sedatives were given. She was able to move about and tend to her regular chores, but was depressed. She takes great pains to indicate, "I never was sorry I was pregnant." However, she was so self-conscious during pregnancy that she would not go out until after dark. She resented financial dependence upon her in-laws.

She had a very difficult time with the delivery, the baby being in transverse position, large (eight pounds at birth) for this small woman; the mother, in addition, was very upset because the obstetrician who was to deliver her was on vacation. No forceps were used, and considerable muscular tearing took place. She was intent on breast feeding the baby despite the position of her in-laws, who felt that the mother's "nervousness" would be transmitted to the baby, if she attempted breast feeding. She was reported by the hospital nurse as "a young, excitable mother." After each nursing the baby vomited, and this symptom was described as typical cyclic vomiting. The child cried a great deal ("sixteen hours out of twenty-four"). Nevertheless, she did not lose weight.

Put on formula after two weeks of breast feeding, the child continued to vomit and often had to take five or six bottles before keeping one down. Then she would quiet down for some time, only to cry again persistently as described above. The infant was "very bright," and her psychomotor development was precocious. She sat up at seven months, said her first word at a year, and spoke short sentences at a year and a half. She walked alone at thirteen months.

This precocious development did not take place in a favorable emotional climate. Reluctantly, the mother brought out that the baby was in an infant home from one to three months of age, because her own condition made it impossible to take care of her. The next five months (3-8 months) the baby was with her grandmother while the mother was in bed with severe colitis. So, actually, prior to eight months of age, the baby was in the mother's care for only the first month of her life. The mother, however resentful of her dependence on her mother-in-law, spent a few months at her in-laws, because she was unable to care for the child herself. She was particularly upset by the fact that the grandmother "acted as if this was her own baby." In later interviews, it was learned that the grandmother became very possessive of the baby, called her variously "our baby" and "my baby," recreating the short-lived experience of her own little girl who had died after six weeks of severe pyloric symptoms. The mother resented the affection given by the grandmother but took pains also to indicate that the child was not happy there either "and had about eight crying spells at bed time." The grandmother was willing to give attention to the baby, holding her about an hour each time until she quieted down. The mother stressed that from birth the child did not seem to be affectionate, even as she reported the closer relation of the baby with the grandmother. When the mother came home with her (ten months), she decided to cut loose from her mother-in-law. She succeeded in keeping the older woman away altogether for eight months. When the baby became acquainted anew with her grandmother who had tended to her for several months, she was hostile toward her and showed no sign of recognition.

The elimination training was initiated by the mother. By virtue of contingencies already described (mother's illness and unsettled home conditions), bladder training was started at twelve months and had been grossly achieved. Bowel training was started earlier (eight months), the grandmother playing the major role and the mother shortly thereafter taking over. The bowel training is not altogether achieved and *smearing* has been continuous until approximately twenty-one months, when it was abruptly interrupted by the type of forceful methods employed when dealing with this young child's "annoying habits." *Rocking* started at approximately fourteen months and is still in evidence. The *pulling of hair* has been referred to. *Thumb sucking*, which greatly disturbed the parents, started at a few weeks. "We didn't do anything about it until three or four months ago." A variety of approaches were then used, which is so often the case when determination backs up the techniques. The child was told she "shouldn't," restriction of movement was applied and a pattern of alternation developed as a result: when one hand was tied, the other was used, one finger in the mouth, one finger in the nose, and the free hand holding the arm involved in

183

the forbidden activity. Note here the flexibility in the alternation of the pattern, which is also characteristic of the very young child. When she was finally subdued in the thumb-sucking activity, she took to *biting herself*. In some way—any way—the tension must be relieved. The child also had *breath-holding spells* which began at about three to four months. "She's had them right along but worse lately." Passing reference is made to the *temper tantrums* and *nightmares* already reported. She has only recently developed specific fears, which again is characteristic of the evolution of early anxiety. She fears moving objects, paper blown by the wind, and some animals.

Almost every function has been involved in the expression of anxiety, and the digestive tract does not escape. She has been a *poor eater*, erratic in her appetite, and at intervals has been given a tonic for the improvement of the latter. The mother volunteers that she sees no connection between external events and her eating difficulties.

Contact with the child: Both parents brought Elly, her father carrying her screaming and her mother at his side looking helpless. This joint session, at the outset seemingly doomed to be fruitless, brings into focus inter-familial relationships as the previous interview could not have. Granted, the mother was to an extent unable to cope with or even hold in her arms this screaming, kicking, at times rigid little body. It was obvious, as time went on, that the father had been more closely associated with this little girl than the mother herself. She clung to him for the major portion of the interview and would not play with toys except when sitting on his lap.

She is a well-developed, well-nourished child, tall for her age, very alert, extremely tense and anxious. The father is easy-going with the child, handles her gently. The three enter the playroom, the child most of the time close to her father and a good deal of this on his lap. At intervals she walks from one to the other parent with her eyes closed, as if to exclude the outside world, a mannerism which is fairly frequently observed in young or very young children who, when they feel that they cannot cope with pressures from the outside, shut the world out with a sign of rejection.

At the beginning, every time she turns, inadvertently or intentionally, toward the writer, she screams anew. The writer makes comments about the little girl who is very scared of this new lady and offers toys, placing them on the table at the child's level. Comments are also made on the little toy people and their relationships, "mommy, daddy, little girl, etc." Very quietly with her eyes closed the child takes possession of several dolls, whispering softly about their identity. She brings her father into all her activities, asking him to hold dolls or help her in the use of crayons. Her productions are mostly of the scribbling type, but her whispering indicates concern with "mommy, daddy, little girl" (not echolalia). It was difficult during this interview to cope with the mother's pressure of speech. She recalled loudly episodes involving herself and her mother-in-law. For instance, she alluded to suicidal threats without suicidal attempt, to anger which could be so violent that "it was frightening," and gave accounts of the dead "pyloric baby."

The child gains a little confidence in the course of the interview, and while she doesn't leave her father's lap, she includes the writer in her play with dolls, her eyes open, she smiles to her, and as she leaves spontaneously says "bye, bye."

Defining the emotional problem: It is obvious that we have here a severely disturbed child—a child whose anxiety is overwhelming and must find expression in disturbed forms of behavior thus far misunderstood and not accepted by her parents. In that age group, anxiety expressions (symptoms) are fluid and interchangeable. We have seen, for instance, that when the child was "slapped out of her tantrum," she took to self-biting. Symptom choice is sometimes clearly legible, as is revealed in information received at a later date about the night disturbances. It was learned that the child was taken to the infant's home *in the evening.* Similarly, when she went to her grandmother's home, it was also *at night,* because her father had to take her after work. Night and bed time, always associated with the interruption of consciousness, temporary death, and an abandonment by the love object, becomes here laden with overwhelming anxiety. It has meant in the realistic past the loss of the mother and is endowed again and again with the threat of this loss.

The child throughout these very traumatic experiences remains in contact with reality. One might ask why, in the face of grave maternal deprivation, this child did not develop more severe symptoms and, in particular, did not become depressed—nor did she withdraw. The answer must be found in two facts: one of an entirely psychological nature, the fact that the grandmother gave her love and warmth, however mis-motivated this may have been; the other, physiological in appearance, the occurrence of cyclic vomiting which was present virtually from birth onwards. The symptoms manifested soon after birth are indicative of a tonicity and excitability which is, for instance, never found in children with early contact disturbances (early infantile autism), nor in infants with depressive symptoms. They are part of the infant's make-up at birth (constitutional) and reveal a readiness to fight back. The defense against anxiety in such a child is attack and aggression.

Briefly, to comment on subsequent therapeutic contacts as they bear on the understanding of the psychodynamics; a few sessions with the parents brought marked changes in the child's behavior and considerable release of her anxiety and tensions. Because of distances travelled, psychotherapy of the child could not be considered by the writer, and a search of local facilities was initiated. The urgency of the child's needs for immediate interpretation of her behavior, the fact that she was troubled, in a sense, ill, was brought out to the parents: not a bad child, but a child in need of comfort, reassurance, and affection.

Shortly after this, she was referred to a mental health clinic in the community. She was in treatment there for a few months. A follow-up inquiry indicated that she was in treatment "for problems of insecurity and problems of relationship with the mother . . . discharged as improved" (clinic report one year later). Three years after the first contact a second follow-up indicated that the mother had placed a request for the reopening of the case, but that the child could not be accepted, because of redistricting rules. It can be assumed that, even in the presence of improved home conditions, unless this child has had intensive psychotherapy she can be expected at this date (age fourteen and a half) to have severe problems of unresolved anxiety.

Reference has been made to the choice of symptom, and the case of a twenty-two-month-old girl briefly to be sketched is given as an illustration. The mother's first statement was, "The child is afraid to go to the bathroom, I think." Still wearing diapers, she was not bowel-trained. The mother reported that she started bowel training at eight months, "catching her." Occasionally the child moved her bowels under such circumstances, but on the whole has not responded to training. The bladder training was started at eight months and had been achieved at thirteen or fourteen months, when a dramatic episode took place which the mother did not bring to light until some time later. The mother made the point that she is "getting practically hysterical if you try to put her on the toilet."

As described here, the child's problem did not reflect the severity of the anxiety and conflict which were later recognized. The mother was bringing her child for observation, because of faulty training, not because she had been sensitive to any emotional disturbance in her child. One of her early comments, indeed, reveals this insensitivity. "I think she's slighting me, she has a look in her eyes." In passing, this is by no means a rare instance, for many parents have difficulty in projecting themselves into a child's emotional world, having repressed many of their own childhood experiences. As this mother does, they interpret the child's behavior as if he or she were twenty-two years old, not twenty-two months.

Bare essentials of the background of both families are given. The paternal grandfather, who made a poor adjustment to his family and to his work, is bitterly resentful of being a failure. The father (twenty-nine years old) lost his mother when sixteen, and must have been very close to her, since he would not talk to his stepmother, nor would he talk about his own mother, considering her memory "sacred," appearing more shy and detached following her death. On the maternal side the grandparents appear better adjusted, with a dominant grandfather and a grandmother who is extremely shy. The father was an only child for a number of years, the only sibling being a girl born of his father's second marriage. A college graduate, he has not made a success of his work. Trained as a chemist, he was at the time of referral working in a factory.

The parents knew each other for ten years before marriage, "but in all that time no knowledge of each other." The marriage has been fraught with many difficulties, some of them originating in the fact, not altogether clear in its motivation, that they were married secretly. The open motivation is that they contributed to the financial support of his family and the father dared not at any time mention the possibility of marrying. Six months after their marriage the father broke with his family altogether, thus stirring up the paternal grandfather's antagonism. "With him it was all or nothing, so we decided nothing." The relations with the father's family have not been resumed. For about one year, the young people lived with the maternal grandparents, after their marriage had been made known to both families.

The mother, twenty-six, is the elder of two children (the second a brother). She acknowledges what she calls "a tendency to be neurotic," listing her many symptoms. Of great significance is the fact that as both young people settled with the mother's parents, she "became quite ill, not physically . . . all diseases . . . so I couldn't work." At the end of the year the maternal grandfather had a coronary thrombosis. "As my father became ill, I recovered." The parents insist that they have been happy in their marriage, but later information brings out different shadings on their married life. The mother described an ambivalent relation to her father, who was nagging and teasing her, but to whom she was very close. She was also very close to her brother—apparently closer to these two men than to her husband. Since her marriage upon graduation from college, she has found compensation for the deficiency through emotional satisfaction in intellectual pursuits. The child was born "three and a half to four years after marriage." The mother obviously was not ready for motherhood, and describes herself as coming back from the hospital "terribly frightened." She has been preoccupied with the thought that "a neurotic mother can only have a neurotic child. . . . I don't want her to be as unhappy as I am." As a young mother she "was . . . not the conventional mother . . . didn't beam." She is obviously formulating her lack of readiness for the motherhood experience. During her pregnancy she had not been happy and had had nausea "most of the time." She became angered easily.

Labor was long and a very frightening experience: myopic and unable to see without her glasses, she was lost when they were taken away from her. She was also given ether either in too large a quantity or was unable to tolerate it. When she became cyanotic, anaesthesia was interrupted, "so I was awake and in pain all the time." Her rejection of the child is made clear in her following statement. "The whole business is a bad thought. I'd like to adopt the next baby. My husband says no. I love my baby but I don't feel it's my own flesh and blood. If I went to a nursery and picked a child I liked, okay." As will shortly be seen, maternal rejection, unspoken though it may be, has its immediate price in the first months of the baby's life.

The infant, put at the breast, had soon to be weaned because of nipple lacerations which were followed by infection —this requiring nearly a year's treatment. The baby, six pounds, five ounces at birth, thrived on the formula and has not been a feeding problem. She slept well, was sociable, her psychomotor development was normal on the early side, with language development somewhat precocious. She has sucked her thumb consistently. The child still sleeps in the parents' bedroom, and the mother sees no untoward effects of the proximity of their marital life to the child. "It hasn't bothered *me*. She's asleep."

The problem for which the child was brought for observation is very definitely localized. At this point it centers on the urinary function. However, the mother reported that shortly before, the child started to *blink* when spanked for what she construed as "bad behavior," i.e., screaming at the peak of urinary retention. Here, again, we see that the blocking of anxiety, without fail, brings in more complex, more remotely related, and less legible manifestations. Blinking may be associated, as often is the case, with shutting out the forbidden (recall mother's statement regarding sleeping conditions).

On the whole, the mother has been attentive to the child's

189

emotional needs. She gave up her work to devote herself to her care, and there is evidence of many small, thoughtful activities devised by her for the child's pleasure—activities which were shared: park outings, visits to mothers with young children, etc. Why the mother showed such irritability through the child's bladder training must obviously be sought in conflicts of her own. The dynamics are not available to the writer, although they were probably later clarified in the course of the mother's analytic therapy. Suggested at the outset, psychoanalytic therapy was postponed because of a long physical illness of the mother and initiated approximately a year and a half later.

The point of interest to us is the background in which the symptoms appeared. As can readily be understood, total significant data are not obtained in the initial interview. Subsequently, however, the mother told of a chance encounter in the park with a man she had been in love with during her college years. He had spurned her, and the marriage with her present husband took place shortly thereafter. The child was fourteen months old and bladder training was a recent achievement when the decisive incident took place. At no time had the mother linked one with the other until inquiry was made into the setup in which the symptoms appeared. She recalled that the little girl had wanted to go to the bathroom, and immediately after the brief encounter she had taken her to a public toilet where she had her first anxiety panic at the time of the flushing. Previous to this, she had been only mildly apprehensive and clung to her mother while being held over adult toilet seats.

Following this episode, the child's behavior was alarmingly altered. For many hours she would control her need to urinate (prolonged urine retention) and cry in fear. To indicate her need she would repeatedly walk toward the bathroom, then refuse to go in, and finally—sometimes after as long as eighteen or twenty hours—she would collapse on the threshold of the bathroom and flood her pants and the floor. This behavior, incidentally, was clearly demonstrated in the playroom at the time of the first session.

The reader will recall that the dramatic episode and its significance were not related initially by the mother, and that the complaint was given as one of faulty training. Following the park incident a series of physical examinations was given, including a cystoscopy, until some pediatrician along the line suggested emotional disturbance as a possible cause.

Not always is the symptom choice of the anxiety as clearly defined. The determining factors in the selection of the organ to be charged with internal tension is often not so easily understood. The complexity of associations, the overlaying of defenses, and the additional traumatizations precipitated by the already existing susceptibility will all concur to render the dynamics less legible.

The immediate outcome of this case is known through a letter received from the mother some twenty months later. As it will be recalled, the mother was then in analytic therapy. This had followed a few sessions with the writer and an additional play session with the child. At that time the little girl was entering a nursery school, and the mother-child relationship had improved considerably.

The two previous cases have illustrated expressions in the young child fairly easily recognized as anxiety. The first one involved almost all somatic and psychological manifestations which can be encountered in that age group. The second pinpointed one facet of symptom-determination.

Anxiety, however, can manifest itself in less direct ways. One of the most common is seen in the *speech and language difficulties* of that age group. Various degrees of *contact disturbances,* the extreme of which is found in early infantile autism, are also worthy of consideration.

Speech and Language Difficulties. As we have seen, this 1 to 3 year age period is decisive in the growth of speech and language. Normal rates and normal forms have been previously examined and their flexibility stressed. There are, however, definite stages which the healthy child must go through. A child who is emotionally deprived or who develops emotional conflict in his relation to his mother may express this conflict by excessive clinging and dependence and hold on to infantile forms of speech expression, may speak little or none at all long after he should have begun. The complete mutism of severe emotional illnesses as schizophrenia is uncommon,

191

but transitory periods of mutism as an emotional disturbance are more frequently encountered.

As a result of the anxiety, infantilism and immaturity of speech are present: elision, substitution of consonants, unduly high pitch, whispered speech, delay in the appearance of sentence structure. Some of the symptomatology listed here is also found in congenital mental retardation. However, the two conditions cannot be confused, if one takes into account the total psychomotor development and analyzes the specific symptoms in terms of total emotional adjustment.

Mild Degrees of Contact Disturbances. As we have seen earlier, the emotionally healthy child gradually develops rapport with the environment, initially through his mother. He shows an interest in the people around him, their actions, their voices, their attention to him, and this interest is in emotional terms. Affective contact is thus recognizable in early life. Severe contact disturbances have already been examined in the light of Spitz's research. His were cases of gross affect disturbances, but all degrees are observable, from mild and transitory apathy and indifference to the extremes found in a disease entity first described by Leo Kanner in 1943.[33]

Early Infantile Autism. Prior to this time, children who presented the clinical picture described by Kanner were usually considered to have congenital mental deficiency, and some of them to be deaf. In his initial paper in 1943 Kanner presented eleven children who showed complete withdrawal of a special type and by 1956 he had studied one hundred and five such children.[34]

Subsequently, Kanner recognized some analogy between the syndrome and early childhood schizophrenia.[35] Nevertheless, early infantile autism stands out as a specific entity with symptoms so characteristic that, once observed, they cannot escape the diagnostic terminology.

The term "early infantile autism" should apply strictly to the syndrome as first described by Kanner. There is a current tendency to apply it to various degrees of autistic behavior which do not, in fact, belong to this definite group.

In his first paper Kanner presented eleven children, eight

boys and three girls (a sex distribution fairly typical of the child population seen in clinics, hospitals, etc., for neurotic and psychotic disorders). Definition centers upon the patients' "inability to relate themselves in the ordinary way to people and situations *from the beginning of life*" (italics mine). The failure of the baby to respond by "anticipatory posture preparatory to being picked up" is the earliest evidence that the child has been unresponsive. In the writer's experience the failure to smile back at the mother at age two to four months is also recorded in these children and is an indication of the same order. While three of the eleven children were mute, eight had spoken at a normal or slightly delayed time. The latter children did not use language "to convey meaning to others."[36] Rote memory is excellent, with "parrot-like repetition of heard word combinations." These word combinations are irrelevant to current situations and often brought out as a kind of "delayed echolalia." Kanner comments on the inflexible meaning of words, their literalness, and the fact that personal pronouns are repeated just as heard. It will be seen that this characteristic usage of personal pronouns is found in the child with early schizophrenia.

He noted that the child's behavior was "governed by an anxiously obsessive desire for the maintenance of sameness." Also typical of these children is the fact that they have good relation to objects and not to persons. This feature is also outstanding in the young schizophrenic's relation to the inanimate and the living. In observing children with early infantile autism one is impressed with the fact that human beings have to them no human quality and can be used, for instance, as chairs to sit on, furniture to push aside, etc. It is clear from their intelligent expression that these children are not retarded. More than that, they reveal observational and retention knowledge, often in great proportions. They are aware of the environment, as indeed is proved when, in the course of therapeutic progress, they are likely, as the young schizophrenics also do, to recall earlier observations and experiences stored up during the incommunicado period. Kanner further comments that they give "an impression of serious-mindedness and, in the presence of others, an anxious tenseness," which is at variance with the appearance of the mentally defective child. They come from intelligent families—not affectionate families—with highly compulsive drives a prominent feature. Physically these children are essentially normal.

In his early communication Kanner established differences between early infantile autism and early schizophrenia on the basis that the symptoms found in the former are at the beginning of life. The extreme aloneness of the autism in the cases he describes begins with birth. The *regression* to withdrawal of young schizophrenics is unlike autistic children's *failure* to establish relationship. As interpreted by Kanner, the latter, to the contrary, may gradually try to enter a world they have never known.

Later, however, Kanner revised his concept of early infantile autism and recognized analogies between the two disease processes. Highlighting the pathognomonic characteristics of the clinical entity he had been first to describe, he wrote in 1949,

> Briefly, the characteristic features consist of a profound withdrawal from contact with people, an obsessive desire for the preservation of sameness, a skillful and even affectionate relation to objects, the retention of an intelligent and pensive physiognomy, and either mutism or the kind of language which does not seem intended to serve the purpose of interpersonal communication. An analysis of this language has revealed a peculiar reversal of pronouns, neologisms, metaphors, and apparently irrelevant utterances which become meaningful to the extent to which they can be traced to the patient's experiences and their emotional implications.[37]

Apart from very minor differences—such as the preservation of sameness, the extreme restrictiveness of their emotional world as seen from the outside, and the affectionate relation to objects, which may be but are not always present in early schizophrenia—the description here given is applicable to the latter syndrome. Indeed, in the same communication Kanner clearly indicated that the basic natures of both entities were so related as to be "indistinguishable" (with special reference to schizophrenia as described by Ssucharewa,[38] Grebelskaya-Albatz,[39] and Despert[40]). However, he also pointed out

194

that the term "insidious onset" would hardly apply to early infantile autism, since the symptomatology is well established toward the end of the first year of life and could thus refer only to the first few months. Recall the earliest indication of the early failure to smile, to assume "anticipatory posture preparatory to being picked up"—both activities representing affective responses to the mother. Kanner came to the conclusion that,

> Early infantile autism may therefore be looked upon as the earliest possible manifestation of childhood schizophrenia. As such, because of the age at the time of the withdrawal, it presents a clinical picture which had certain characteristics of its own, both at the start and in the course of later development.[41]

ADDITIONAL OBSERVATIONS ON EARLY INFANTILE AUTISM:

At the present time enough cases of early infantile autism have been presented, and Kanner's own descriptions have been so full, that there seems no need to bring again a clinical case for total presentation. However, in attempting to clarify the concept, particularly in the aspect of its possible causes, therapeutic experience with fifteen boys and three girls during recent years has brought to light certain facets which may be worthy of description. The writer's experience conforms with that of Kanner as regards the characteristics of the parents, in particular the impersonality and emotional vacuity of the rapport between parent and child. An uncommunicative mother, advised by her therapist to talk *to* her child, is seen putting her baby in the go-cart. She talks *at* the child, enumerating in great detail the different stages of this operation. The child does not look at her, does not listen, remains immobile and untouched under the profusion of language—a language devoid of emotional content. Of the same order is the mechanical quality of the rapport between mother and child when the child is heard enumerating for his or her mother the parts of objects, including face and body of humans present. The human being is viewed and felt, not as one, but as made up of parts. If he is viewed as one, he must remain exactly as first perceived (obsessive wish for maintenance of sameness). A part can be as meaningful as a whole, but actually neither has emotional meaning. Kanner has commented upon this aspect of maintenance of sameness.[42] Many diaries kept by the parents of these children have been read. Never is "our baby" or other equally fond expressions found. It is "the girl . . . the boy . . . he . . . she," and with every turn of the page one expects a reference to "the case."

Also to be noted are the early misinterpretations made by the parents. They reflect in the face of obvious anomalies an absence of outspoken anxiety which is very striking and certainly speaks for a lack of sensitivity to the child's feelings. For instance, one such young child can be viewed as "cheerful" because of his laughing by himself, particularly at night. However, anyone looking at the child would recognize this type of laughter as one without apparent motivation. One who has empathy with infants and who is familiar with their multiple sources of pleasure will recognize the difference. Similarly, obvious and tenacious compulsions are interpreted as being "tidy" or "orderly" like one's mother or father. A child is described as having many accomplishments, having learned to "talk with his fingers . . . talk to his ears." This refers to a compulsive gesture which consists of bringing the thumbs to the ears and moving the other fingers rapidly in the air (one of the large variety of motor compulsions exhibited by this group of children).

Of the same nature (misinterpretation) is the neglect of the infant's great need for body contact and closeness to the mother: the scientific approach with all the hygienic laws observed, the schedule rigidly adhered to, and, in between, no allowance for body nearness. These are the babies who, as diaries show us, are left in their cribs between the feedings, which are at best mechanical. The babies are put in play pens at three to six months, as if expected to entertain themselves and enjoy solitude. *Rocking* during the first two years, and even later sometimes, is a very common manifestation. Twirling, spinning, "winding," and *compulsive handling of objects* has been reported by Kanner and others. Together with other compulsive gestures referred to above they can be interpreted as defenses against the overwhelming anxiety these children experience. Supporting this interpretation is an observation frequently made in the course of therapy, that they may decrease temporarily in a phase where the child is obviously less anxious, and they do eventually disappear when, also in the course of therapy, the child has come to accept compromises between the maintenance of his rigid autistic world and the external reality world.

Mechanical body restraint (splints for congenital foot defects, for instance) is reported in the history of several of these children.

Three more points are worthy of comment: (1) the acuteness of sensory perception encountered in this group; (2) the excellent motor coordination which parallels and is in apparent contradiction with requested motor performances; (3) the positive aspect of the child's determination to maintain his inner world as established and the *determination not to communicate*, both of which are also found in young schizophrenics.

The *acuteness of sensory perception* upon first examination appears to be in contradiction with the lack of response to external stimuli. Indeed, as mentioned, these children almost invariably are first tested for deafness. Upon continued careful observation, however, it is found that these children have an acute perceptiveness in all sensory fields. Several of them have been found to respond to supersonic whistle, i.e., pitches ordinarily not registered by the human ear, and also to low pitch sounds, such as the barely perceptible rumble of an oil furnace starting up. Whether this actually represents more acute perception or greater inner concentration with coincident selective exclusion of undesirable stimuli is not clear.

In the visual field one cannot fail to be impressed with the extraordinary acuteness of perception of a child who, returning to the playroom after several days, will arrange a large number of toys in exactly the same pattern as he had before. If, during a moment of inattention on the part of the child, one such toy is displaced slightly, he quickly discovers it and sometimes goes into a panic as a result. Many of the anxiety reactions which are often at the moment unintelligible to the observer may be the child's reactions to these acute perceptions. For instance, one child suddenly became panicky as he was watching a point in space beyond the window of the office. A slight fluttering of leaves in a nearby tree, barely perceptible to an ordinary observer, proved to be the stimulus. As is often the case, animation of an inanimate object had greatly perturbed the child. This was corroborated when it was possible to bring the child to the tree, touch it, handle its leaves, and generally be reassured. The frequent smelling before handling, the negative and positive reactions to smells of bodies, clothing, etc., the touch perception and the sharp awareness of textures, the tasting and licking as they entail choice or rejection, all indicate an unusual sensitiveness to sensory stimuli.

The *excellent motor coordination* is evident in such activities as the handling of phonograph records so early (one and a half to three years is reported) that an ordinary child of corresponding age would be at a loss to duplicate the performance. The children under discussion, without any group play experience, easily pick up a ball, if they so wish, and play like veteran little leaguers, or else climb a tricycle which they have not used previously and ride with great skill. In their manipulation of toys they reveal the same quality, and not one child has ever shown motor awkwardness. One boy, in a sudden panic, managed literally to climb up a wall for a few steps, a feat for which the human body has not been devised. These motor achievements, while they appear to be of the acquired type, are nevertheless primal, the fluidity of motor action being based not on training but on unhampered and instinctual motor expression (return to earlier forms of motility).

The third point to be emphasized refers to a very positive aspect of the illness under consideration, namely, the *determination of the child to retain his inner world as it is*. One cannot fail to be impressed with the tenaciousness, in so young and necessarily immature a personality structure, of the intensity of this drive. For instance, in the course of therapy a child who has been mute or nearly mute for several years, if impelled spontaneously to use language, will be seen to punish himself (biting, hitting self), even knocking his head against the wall, as it were in punishment against an impulse which disrupts the forces at work in the isolating process.

Definite a clinical picture as it is, early infantile autism remains baffling to the thoughtful observer, particularly with regard to its etiology. The analogy with childhood schizophrenia is well established. However, the development of schizophrenia requires the emergence of the ego in its reality-testing function. Clearly, this emergence is gradual and begins at birth, but at the age where early infantile autism can be recognized, i.e., two to three months, one cannot speak of ego formation, even as the infant at that age is slowly developing an awareness of self as part of and also apart from the mother—the dawn of reality testing. The particular quality —physiological and psychological—in the infant which makes for his failure to respond affectively is unknown. Its background may be a complex admixture of influences, some of which will possibly in the near future be traceable to maternal attitudes during pregnancy. Current investigations of birth conditions as related to maternal attitudes during pregnancy, psychological factors operating in spontaneous abortions, etc., lead the way to an understanding of very complex reactions heretofore neglected.

EARLY INFANTILE AUTISM, THE AUTISTIC CHILDREN, AND AUTISTIC BEHAVIOR:

Since its application to children, the concept of autism has been widely used. Its diffusion has not increased its clarification. On the contrary, in current terminology an "autistic" child may be a child with well-circumscribed or minor autistic manifestations or, at the other extreme, an uncontested case of early infantile autism. Isolated manifestations of autism do not make a case of early infantile autism. For instance, a young child may spend considerable time in twirling objects or in playing out bizarre fantasies, which on first observation are unintelligible. While these fantasies may be in every respect similar to fantasies found in schizophrenia or early infantile autism, if taken out of context, they do not of necessity warrant a diagnosis of infantile autism or early schizophrenia. The affective contact with reality which is present remains the index to make or rule out the diagnosis.

AUTISM AS DEFINED BY BLEULER:

In order better to evaluate the concept of autism and its position in child psychiatry it is necessary to go back to the concept as originally defined by Bleuler. In *Dementia Praecox or the Group of Schizophrenias,* he writes,

> schizophrenia is characterized by a very peculiar alteration of the relation between the patient's inner life and the external world. The inner life assumes pathological predominance (autism). . . . This detachment from reality together with the relative and absolute predominance of the inner life, we term autism. . . . The reality of the autistic world may seem more valid than that of reality itself; the patients then hold their fantasy world for the real, reality for an illusion. They no longer believe in the evidence of their own senses. . . . Wishes and fears constitute the contents of autistic thinking. . . . Autistic thinking obeys its own special laws. . . . Autistic thinking is directed by affective needs; the patient thinks in symbols, in analogies, in fragmentary concepts, in accidental connections. . . . Autism must not be confused with the "unconscious." Both autistic, and realistic thinking can be conscious as well as unconscious.[43]

The autism of adult and childhood schizophrenia is well recognized. The affective contact with reality has been severed. With early infantile autism affective contact with reality fails to be attained. Kanner's description of his cases is explicit on this subject.

SOME CONSIDERATIONS RELATING TO THE GENESIS OF AUTISTIC BEHAVIOR IN CHILDREN:

The term *autistic*, which until recent years applied to certain mental disorders of adulthood, has come more and more to be associated with childhood disorders and even to designate the pathological core of one specific syndrome of infancy and early childhood: early infantile autism, described by Kanner. Since the concept is increasingly included in describing some pathological behavior found in young children, it has seemed appropriate further to scrutinize the concept itself by inquiring into the dynamics of its manifestations.

The case material here presented is offered in an effort to clarify the relation of maternal attitudes to the development of autistic behavior in young children.

A 40-year-old married woman was referred to me for treatment three years ago by a child psychiatrist. The circumstances of this unusual referral of a woman patient from one child psychiatrist to another were as follows: Eight months earlier he had examined this woman's only child, a boy then five years old, and diagnosed him as a case of early infantile autism. This was the final examination in a series of psychiatric examinations which began when the boy was two and a half years old. Following the last period of examination and diagnosis, the child had been placed with a foster family and he was there at the time of the mother's initial contact with me.

The patient was three months pregnant and obsessed with the thought that she could give birth only to an abnormal child, similar to her son in every respect, although she had been assured by the first child psychiatrist that instances of two autistic children in one family had never been known. Her first statement was, "I have a little boy afflicted with a severe emotional difficulty," and thereafter, through the eighteen interviews which preceded the birth of her second child, a girl, she spent considerable time going over the little boy's early years. The number of interviews was limited by the fact that distances travelled were considerable, but her schedule was so arranged that unlimited time could be spent as needed. The material is not presented as chronologically obtained, but time sequences are pointed out when meaningful. The type of therapy applied in this case was mostly supportive, with gentle probing where indicated and interpretations, the depth of which was determined by the degree of emotional readiness and tolerance which the patient demonstrated. A transference was established fairly early in the therapeutic contact, but it could not be described as a very dependent relationship.

After some ineffectual attempts at abortion on the part of the patient, unknown to others, the possibility of a therapeutic abortion had been seriously considered by the family physician, who was alarmed by the patient's rejection of the pregnancy and even more so by her crying spells, sleeplessness, restlessness, and anorexia. However, this had been firmly opposed by her husband, a minister, who said of his wife, "I've never considered anything wrong with her—she has her moments of depression, but who hasn't?" He tended to see "a bit of exhibitionism" in her behavior, but also volunteered the information that he felt at the beginning that "she might harm herself. For a while, I never let her out of my sight." Although he had, and was somewhat boastful of, a considerable experience as a counselor of adolescents, young married couples, and parents in relation to their children, he had no insight into his wife's condition nor any patience with her complaints.

The "sixth or seventh of ten children," the husband, then 45, had reportedly had a happy childhood in spite of rickets, which prevented his walking until the age of four. He was very close to his remaining five brothers and sisters, all of whom were successful in their respective professions. He was himself brilliant, outgoing, optimistic, a man of vigorous intellect and insatiable drive for activity. He had made a success not only of his church work but also of a variety of social and religious causes, into which he threw himself wholeheartedly and which he supported with indefatigable energy. He had expected his wife to become actively associated with his church and its social activities, and in that he had been disappointed. It is interesting to note that when seen jointly with his wife in the final interview long after their baby girl was born, in response to my suggestion that his wife needed and would wish treatment for herself, he expressed the wish for a personal analysis so that he might become a better counselor. To sum it up, although he was outwardly warm and friendly, the compulsiveness, rigidity and egocentricity of his personality seemed well established.

Although this husband had been fleetingly aware of the

possibility of his wife's self-destruction, while the several physicians who had seen her thought of her as a suicidal risk and the patient herself frequently stated that she was "depressed, nervous, and unhappy," I never feared suicide since there seemed to be no indications of self-destructive drives as revealed in direct statements, dreams, fantasies, or her attitudes toward marriage and motherhood. The predominant mood was never in the nature of a true depression; for while she ruminated over her personal misfortunes, her way of dealing with them always revealed aggression turned toward the environment rather than toward herself.

The patient was an attractive woman, superficially pleasant and smiling, with a tendency toward childish mannerisms and ways of verbal expression, in spite of a broad culture and extensive intellectual interests. She was reluctant to give her age, emphasizing, "I don't like to tell and acknowledge that I'm middle-aged." She was the sixth of ten children (5 boys, self, boy, 3 girls) and had spent the major part of her life, until her marriage at 22, in a small town in a southern state. She insisted that her childhood years had been happy, that she was babied and overindulged by her parents and five older brothers; but much of her childhood experience was blocked and distorted, as revealed, for instance, in her account that when a little girl, although bathing daily with her older brothers, she "yet was never aware of their sex organs." When at some time I pointed out that her attitude toward childbirth (to be elaborated upon) must have been colored by her mother's numerous pregnancies, she recalled that at seven, knowing that another baby was expected, she had asked her mother where it would come from and was told that it would come in the doctor's bag. "I must have been suspicious because I said, 'Why doesn't he smother?' Then I remember saying quickly, 'Probably because the doctor comes so fast he doesn't have time to smother.'" She insisted that there was a great deal of security in the family and that she never heard her mother "grumbling" about having so many children. "Maybe that's why I didn't notice she was deformed." She felt that she was given a good start in her family but she "always lacked a certain sense of inner direction." This refers to a certain emotional detachment which she experienced early in life and which she frequently contrasted with her husband's closeness to his own family and other people. The detachment and emotional blurring were apparent in her accounts of college life and vague plans of becoming a teacher (she was briefly a substitute teacher). At 22 she married her present husband and moved to a small community in a northern state, where her husband was a minister. For the first time she was away from home (the college she attended was in her home town). She was lonely and wanted her parents to visit her and help her make the adjustment. Her mother deliberately refused to come to see her for almost three years. "I had to change from a school girl to a minister's wife." Her husband was out of the home a good deal, and she "hated" to go along with him to meetings, church parties, etc. She attempted to do some volunteer social work but turned back rather quickly to reading in isolation, retaining a minimum social contact in the congregation. When her husband gave her little sympathy, she felt the fault was her own inadequacy rather than any lack of understanding on his part.

Information regarding her sexual adjustment was obtained in the course of several interviews as a result of investigating her attitude toward childbirth, which she had from the start strongly qualified in negative terms. It must be recalled at this point that all probing into her earlier experiences always had to be started from the feelings she expressed about her first child, since she was so obsessively preoccupied with him. However, her feeling toward childbirth, expressed in the first interview, was unequivocal. "It's so messy! Revolting! A child's birth to me is barbarous—never do I want to hear the word 'push!' I was exhausted, couldn't understand how such a beautiful baby could be born out of filth and slime."

The first child was born after twelve years of marriage, as a result of a slip in contraceptive methods (*coitus interruptus* and wife's preventive preparations). Labor was long, 24 hours, but there were no complications. Although it was not until the sixth interview that she began to question her sexual adjustment ("I hope I won't discover that I am a frigid woman"), one can anticipate to report that she did not experience any orgasm until after the birth of her second child, that is, after eighteen years of marriage. The first sexual contact was painful and several months after her marriage she consulted a physician, who examined her and reported her as being still a virgin, and advised her to relax. Two years later she consulted a gynecologist who performed a vaginal dilation. Two or three years later she consulted a birth-control clinic and one more gynecologist. She felt from the start that she was afraid of pregnancy, but she later reasoned that that could not be the only explanation as she found that while pregnant she experienced the same fear. She was sure she loved her husband, and not only in a platonic way, but she was at a loss to understand her feeling toward sex. ("I close up and reject my husband. I do not know how I could ever become pregnant.")

Although she continued to think of childbirth as "a horrible business," she was never conscious of rejecting her child, and she set to work at the bringing up of "the perfect child." Her description of the perfect bringing up included the rigid enforcement of rules regarding the sterilization of bottles, the feeding schedule, etc. ("They told me in the hospital that I shouldn't feed the baby at 2 A.M. I let him cry.") She followed literally the advice of her pediatrician (at least what she interpreted as his advice) when he said, "Don't pick up your baby." Her husband was not allowed in the baby's room without first changing his clothes, washing his hands thoroughly, and so on, lest he should bring in germs. Furthermore, she objected to what seems to have been a very natural desire on the part of the father to handle and fondle the baby. ("I couldn't stand my husband around the child.") That she excluded all others in the family and took possession of the child is clear from her descriptive statement: "I thought, 'I'm going to raise me a nice child.' After he was born, he seemed the perfect child for me." He was indeed a very good baby; and while caring for him, she entertained not vague fantasies but specific pictures of what he was to become.

Her devotion as a mother seems to have found expression entirely in the mechanical and rigid furthering of dietary and hygienic measures. The absence of mothering and fondling of the child and her inability to enjoy body contact with her baby are revealed in very significant statements, as "I can't have a child swarm all over me; I have to be by myself to relax." Even when she was expecting the baby, she could not think of him as an infant. "I had to look forward to when he'd be five or six years old. I wanted a child who could tell me something." A reported comment from her friends throws a light on the lack of relatedness of this mother to her child. "They said I look more natural with a book under my arm than with a baby in a carriage. Why should I look natural? I didn't feel natural."

Although the child's psychomotor development was normal, even in some respects precocious, he never attempted to communicate, was more interested in musical records and calendars than in people. Head banging, temper tantrums, thumb sucking, and nail biting, all attacked by the mother with varying determination, came and went. When placed in a nursery school at three years, the child was dry, but he was consistently enuretic at home until 4½. Similarly, when placed in a hospital for a six months' observation period at four years, he ate well, but he always had feeding difficulties at home.

To sum up, this young woman was compulsive, perfectionistic, narcissistic, immature, frigid, emotionally detached, frightened by body contact, lacking in sensuousness, and capable of functioning satisfactorily only on an intellectual level. Her first child was a clear-cut case of early infantile autism.

In attempting to clarify this woman's attitude toward sex, as she was elaborating on her "ideal" childhood, I pointed out that there seemed to be some discrepancy between her reportedly blissful experiences in a family of ten children and her subsequent rejection of the sexual side of marriage and motherhood. The patient said at first that she might have felt the disappointment of her mother in some of her children. This seemed a very superficial rationalization, and this was pointed out to her with the comment that further back, in her early years, there might have been some experiences which were instrumental in shaping her attitude of revulsion toward sex. Shortly thereafter she brought up a memory, which had undoubtedly been very close to consciousness, relative to a traumatic episode which had taken place when she was approximately four years old. A cousin, thirteen or fourteen years old, apparently attempted sexual intercourse with her. "He tried to rape me. I remember being naked, or partly naked. I don't remember any sex thrill." For a whole year she was terrified by him because he would watch for opportunities to be alone with her, and he made at least two similar attempts. One year after the first episode he was killed in a hunting accident, and she remembered feeling "glad when he died because he was bad anyway." She had felt guilty over such a reaction and elaborated a confused fantasy regarding sex, rape and illegitimate children, which was not helped by her mother's repeated warnings about men bothering little girls, and also her awareness that her mother's watchfulness during her preadolescent years was in some definite way connected with her own fear. Her comments regarding the sexual attempts are self-explanatory. "I have never gotten over my resentment—it seems rather simple, yet it must be significant, it was so ugly—maybe something happened that made me close, even though my husband is sexually attractive and he certainly didn't try to rape me."

She was last seen, before the birth of the baby, about one month before the anticipated date of delivery. Although there can be no question of fundamental change in her personality, change was nevertheless accomplished in that her tenseness and obsessive thinking were at a minimum and that she looked toward the event of delivery with what she called "at least some peace of mind." That this was accomplished on the basis of transference, with the therapist in the role of the mother figure, is clearly legible in a letter written a few days before her admission to the hospital. "You have helped me a great deal and I hope you won't be disappointed in me." Being fully aware that no fundamental change could have been brought about, I had stressed the need, in helping this mother plan for the bringing up of the baby, of the mother's being relieved of most of the chores attached to formulas and schedules. The parents agreed to hire a full-time nurse, and this plan was carried out for several months. The mother was not seen during this period, in part because distances were a definite handicap, but mainly because the father, now relieved of his anxiety regarding his wife's condition, saw no purpose in continued contacts. However, she wrote to me fairly regularly, giving the homey small details which help build a remote clinical picture. A week after the birth of the baby girl, she wrote that she had experienced a short, normal labor and delivery, adding, "My normal experience with child-birth this time has greatly helped me." She had a sense of accomplishment about her part in it and referred to being proud of herself. She must also have experienced consider-able relief and a measure of deep gratification in her new experience of motherhood, for she wrote, "I am feeling hap-pier than I have for years," a statement which she reiterated in another letter two months later. The baby was reported then as smiling, cooing, responsive and developing normally. The mother, still preoccupied with the other child, was mak-ing comparisons between the two, expressing no concern over the little girl but engaging in many wishful fantasies about the little boy. She identified the girl with her first child to the extent that she sometimes called her by his name. She ex-pressed the wish to return for continued therapy, but her husband was violently opposed to it, emphasizing once more his belief (also expressed to me at the outset) that her whole trend of obsessive thoughts about the second pregnancy and the future of the second baby had been initiated by the sug-gestion of a physician. The father's interpretation of this sug-gestion was that the physician implied that if she were not treated, her baby might be like her first child, an interpreta-tion which carried no supportive evidence.

When the baby was four months old, the mother, who had temporarily lost her nursemaid, wrote a letter in which the first sign of anxiety appeared. She was overwatchful of the baby, who until then had been nursed in a relaxed, easy atmosphere. If the baby did not cry for a period of time, the mother felt she was "too good" and promptly set about stim-ulating her. How this was done was not indicated. It was not until one month later (baby then five months) that the mother could be seen. Owing to severe weather conditions the baby could not be brought in, and the father was even reluctant to let his wife come in. Detailed questioning and the pe-rusal of several photographs clearly indicated that the baby was a healthy, cheerful, responding baby; she was not on a schedule and the parents were evidently more "relaxed" about her than they had been with the little boy. "We haven't had an argument about this baby as we did with him, all the time." Her preoccupation with the boy, though not so obsessive, was still interfering with her enjoyment of the new baby, and on two occasions she had dashed South to visit him. She was quite ambivalent toward the foster parents, especially the mother, for whom the boy, now 6½, had formed a close attachment and dependence. There was one more disturbing element in the family besides the absence of a nursemaid, namely, the fact that the paternal grandmother had settled with them. This had necessitated a considerable readjustment of personalities and even of the residential setup. It was again strongly emphasized that efforts should be made to find at least a partial mother-substitute. It was in the course of this interview that the mother reported that she had experienced orgasm for the first time in her life, following the birth of the baby and after eighteen years of marriage. "I don't suppose he feels so henpecked now that he can dominate me sexually."

Letters continued to come in, reporting normal progress in the child including emotional response and speech development, but when the child was sixteen months old the question came up for the first time between the parents regarding the need for a direct checkup. At this time, however, the parental motivation showed a divergent orientation. The father was urging the mother to have a psychiatric examination of the child, not because of any concern he might have about her, but to "put an end once and for all" to the mother's anxiety. The mother, on the other hand, was now reluctant to bring in the child because of her own "unhappy associations and recollections of these tests and interviews with pediatricians and psychologists, etc." The mother's attitude was the more remarkable as she was the one to be so anxious about the child, whom she reported in her letter as "less sociable." The pediatrician expressed no concern over the baby's development then. Weather conditions upstate made travel difficult, and once more the checkup was postponed.

It was not until five months later, the child being then 21 months old, that the mother, then the child, and finally both

209

parents were seen in rapid succession. The mother was tense; she cried with a depth of feeling which had not been in evidence before. "I couldn't face it a second time." She reported that the child still communicated clearly and relevantly for her needs, but that she had gradually lost interest in people, children or adults, with whom she had previously been friendly, and she did not respond to them as in the past. She had been playing normally with a baby girl, six months younger than herself, but was now easily frightened by her; and if this child cried, she would run away from her, screaming. She screamed a good deal, mostly when frustrated, for instance, when her mother was not entirely attentive to her. The father made constant comparisons with this apparently better-adjusted little neighbor and had become very anxious himself. He said to the mother, "You know we're not good parents; it's affected our child." There was no rigidity in their planning for the child, and they had no open arguments. However, a revealing comment was made: "We're very tense; we're at her all the time, always testing her. We push her; when I quit it my husband goes on with it." The pediatrician consulted shortly before had observed the child at length and summarized his suggestions with the brief recommendation: "Quit taking her emotional temperature." Although the mother described their sexual adjustment as "better than ever before," their relation as parents had deteriorated, owing to increased tension between them and the father's insistence that his wife was responsible for recent developments. In anger he had told her, "Before you do anything further to this child, we're going to board her; you're not going to kill her like you did her brother." The father, seen during the last part of this interview, threw additional light on the mother's ambivalence of feeling. Clarifying the circumstances which had caused the mother to be in full charge most of the time, contrary to suggestions, he said that several times when they had been able to secure a full-time nursemaid, the mother would accept and then at the last moment reject her. She wanted to take care of the baby yet "resents the care." At this point, the mother said explosively, "Yes, sometimes I resent her (the child)." She had become aware of her rejection of this child as well as of the first one. In the two-year interval there had taken place a marked change in the father's personality. He had grown old, bitter, and intolerant of his wife.

The child, seen a few days later, was an attractive, alert little girl. She had come with both parents and clung to her father, who, though tender and loving, seemed also helpless and passive with her. Without much difficulty she came to the playroom with her mother. At first clinging to her and whining without tears, she began to explore the room without touching anything, her eyes wandering about with a solemn, preoccupied expression, no smile, no external manifestation of anxiety, about the unfamiliar person and environment. She used a few single words appropriately, as related to her parents, toys, etc. Once when she wanted to see her father, she took her mother's hand and led her to the door, saying softly, "Daddy." She responded, not consistently but at intervals, to my affectionate approaches and suggestions for play. Several times, as the mother was not quick to satisfy her request for her total attention, she threw herself on the floor screaming, face down. She spontaneously chose, and engaged in at length, a type of compulsive play which consisted of rolling a car back and forth, hundreds of times, over the marble sill of the bathroom door, all the while muttering to herself something about "car," completely ignoring her mother and me. A very revealing incident took place which crystallized, for the observer, the mother-child relationship. The little girl had climbed on her mother's lap obviously for a little cuddling, and the mother was holding her at arm's length, both of them in rigid motor attitudes, while the baby pointed to each of the mother's facial features, giving softly the appropriate name, singsong, in the best old-fashioned classroom manner. There was a lack of spontaneity and emotional response in the mother and a robotlike mechanical character to the relationship. This was undoubtedly a very disturbed child who reacted to an intolerable situation by withdrawing, a situation in which tender, emotional gratification from the mother was unavailable, while tremendous pressures for intellectual growth and achievements were exerted by both parents. The reactions were not irreversible, and the child was capable of responding to an affectionate approach

211

from others in the environment. While a diagnosis of infantile autism would not be warranted, there was every indication that the child's emotional development was in the direction of schizophrenic-like patterns. It was felt that, even at the cost of family disruption, radical changes should be made if a psychotic development were to be averted; a mother-substitute to take charge and the mother to be treated. Despite their expressed partial awareness, further resistance from both parents was encountered. I did not hesitate, however, to depict the child's future rather forcefully as an "either-or" situation, the need for a warm, simple, perhaps uneducated but child-loving nursemaid being particularly stressed.

Fortunately, it was found possible to refer the family to a child guidance clinic which had begun to function in their locality. While intensive therapy could not be carried out, both the mother and child were seen individually, at two-week intervals, by a psychiatrist who, five months later, reported "a definite improvement" in the child's adjustment, commenting particularly that while the child "still smiles rarely when unobserved, her responses to gentle social stimulation are becoming more adequate." While the psychotherapeutic work, however limited in time, must have played a part, the psychiatrist writes, "I think the nursemaid, a pleasant, middle-aged woman who has taken care of the child . . . deserves full credit for the positive change. She is loving and quiet with the child. . . ."

The mother had difficulties at first in accepting the nurse, but significantly wrote some months later that she was happy to see that the child was becoming more affectionate toward her (the mother) as a result. In reporting on her child's progress and the happier relation between the parents, she stressed the fact that her own anxiety had been allayed by the assurance from the two psychiatrists about "the normalcy of our daughter" (that is, that she was not another case of infantile autism).

During the past three years, 46 mothers of 33 boys and 13 girls, under twelve years of age, presenting severe emotional, intellectual, and behavior manifestations characteristic of a schizophrenic process, have come to my attention. The case just presented was selected because the mother's personality structure is fairly representative of the group and also because of the unusual opportunity this case offered to study a mother-child relationship in the making and to obtain knowledge of its dynamics.

Such opportunities are rare, owing to the type of resistance encountered in these mothers; as a rule it is difficult to secure a dynamically meaningful picture of maternal attitudes, as would be the case with mothers of neurotic children (note the many studies of mothers of anxious, stuttering, compulsive children, etc.). They reject treatment for themselves; and when it is possible to link them actively to the therapeutic process, their participation remains one of contribution to the child's treatment rather than any involvement in their own personal difficulties. They see the problem outside of themselves; they are victims of, rather than contributors to, the misfortune that has befallen them. This is clearly seen, for instance, in the Bellevue report on the treatment program for parents of schizophrenic children.[45] The parents, and especially the mother, are very articulate regarding their confusion, their guilt reactions, their inability to identify with their child, and the hostility he brought out in them. Although it is reported that they felt responsible for their child's illness, that they had scrutinized their own background and their handling of the child, there is no indication that they revealed the kind of persons that they themselves were, the kind of emotional and sexual adjustment they themselves had made. It is also interesting to note that maternal attitudes are sometimes presented as resulting from the child's illness, rather than as psychogenetically linked to it. Bender, for instance, writes: "The mother of the schizophrenic child, especially the child in whom the process has developed insidiously over a long period, shows a specific mechanistic patterning due to her efforts to help the child in his distorted identification process, to understand what is happening and to identify herself with the child."[46]

In a few publications found in the literature[47, 48, 49] studies of mothers of schizophrenic children and adults show a large measure of agreement on characteristic maternal attitudes. A pertinent summarized description from Tietze[50] is quoted: "All mothers were overanxious and obsessive, all were domineering. . . . All mothers were found to be restrictive with regard to the libidinal gratification of their children. Most of them were perfectionistic and oversolicitous and more dependent on approval by others than the average mother. . . ."

Kanner,[51] in reporting on autistic disturbances of affective contact in children, refers to the high intelligence and obsessiveness of the parents. He also comments: "In the whole group, there are very few really warm-hearted fathers and mothers. . . . Even some of the happiest marriages are rather cold and formal affairs."

In the studies which appear in the literature, the mothers of schizophrenic children or adults were seen when the illness was already well established, so that however carefully the mother-child relationship might be evaluated, it would be difficult to dissociate the primary maternal attitude from secondary reactions, that is, the complex psychological reactions set up in the mother by the child's abnormal behavior.

It is sometimes also argued that these mothers had other children who were normal or relatively normal, but it must be remembered that a mother, biogenetically identical for all her children, may nevertheless psychogenetically differ widely from one child to the other. In the case described here, it is clearly seen that the mother of the second child was not identical with the mother of the first, even while acknowledging that no considerable change was effected through therapy. Variations in the primary maternal attitude take on an additional significance when looked at from the point of view of ordinal position; and the fact that 39 of the 46 children in the group were either first in line or only children cannot be ignored.

The question which must be asked is, "What is the meaning of this particular child to this particular mother?" In the case under discussion, it is clear that the first child (the boy with the diagnosis of early infantile autism) was not only rejected, as rejection is generally understood, but was also involved in a conflict which made sex powerfully tabooed and childbirth in a sense illegitimate (recall the involved fantasy regarding sex, rape, and illegitimacy). The sensuous pleasures associated with infant care, which mothers usually reveal in indirect statements in their accounts of the baby's first year, are here forbidden. In the light of her own traumatic sexual experience at three or four years, it is interesting to note that she could not visualize her child until the age of 5 or 6, as if her identification with the baby made it compulsory for her to blot out his early years. Although no deep analysis of this mother's sexual conflict was made, the nature of the conflict, even in its more superficial aspects, is so significant that conclusions regarding its bearing on the rejection of motherhood are inescapable.

The pioneering work of Ribble[52] and Spitz[53] has opened the way to a deeper understanding of the mother-infant interrelationship. Both have in particular reported on the devastating effects that the removal of the mother has on the infant's emotional balance and growth. An analysis of the qualities of mothering as they are so pointedly described by Ribble must necessarily lead back to the mother's own sexual adjustment. The fact that so many mothers of these children are emotionally detached and seeking gratification from intellectual sources rather than from contact with people should be emphasized in this connection. Kanner,[54] has stated, "My search for autistic children of unsophisticated parents has remained unsuccessful to date"; and indeed if the parents do not all find their way into the "Who's Who of Science," it can be said that many of the mothers surround their infant with a scientific aura and emotional void which are very striking; they are proud of the "objectivity" they have shown, they frequently refer to "observing" their children as though they were clinical subjects, they compile detailed notes and diaries on them, they apply literally the rigid and mechanistic rules which they are quick to seize upon as ways and means of rearing the perfect child.

It is doubtful if the sense of guilt about forbidden sexual and sensuous expression can be seen so clearly operating in all cases as in the case here described, and there are probably as many forms of motivation as there are individuals. However, the question can be raised in view of two significant characteristics of the mother and child which are frequently encountered in the group, namely, the emotional detachment

and the overintellectualization in the mother and the early
absorption of the child in nonhuman content and nonfunc-
tional activities, such as extensive acquisition of knowledge
of musical records, license plate numbers, astronomical data,
large and inappropriate vocabulary, word spelling, etc. On the
one hand, the mother is remote and, as expressed by Tietze,
"restrictive to the libidinal gratification" of her child; and on
the other she puts excessive pressure on the growing baby to
achieve feats of development which are considerably beyond
his age level and interests. The core of the pathological problem in all the children is a disturbance of contact with reality
which may be noted in some during the first months of life.
For many of them, there have been lacking the warmth, the
closeness, the body contact pleasures from the mother, which
are recognized as essential to a normal development of relation to reality. How early is the infant developing a sense
of separateness from its mother? How is normal detachment achieved? One can speculate on the questions, but certainly the problem of affective contact with reality in the
young child must hinge upon the kind of satisfactions or
frustrations experienced by the infant in his early dependency
on his mother.

EMOTIONAL DISTURBANCES OF THE THREE
TO SIX YEAR PERIOD

New forms of emotional disturbances appear during this
period. They are of three main types: *disturbances of verbal
communication, of social relationships and behavior,* and,
finally, *disturbances marked by compulsions* in a variety of
patterns. The fact that the superego emerges during this period gives direction to the symptomatology.

Anxiety manifestations as noted in the earlier period are
also encountered, but defenses against the anxiety which
could not appear prior to superego development now put in
an appearance. At this time one can speak of anxiety neurosis
or anxiety state. *Disturbances of contact* (schizophrenia), usually identified at a later date, have, in a number of cases,
their onset during this age period. *Psychosomatic manifestations* are rare outside of simple disfunctions (anorexia, in-

somnia, gastro-intestinal disturbances, etc.), and *hypochondriacal complaints* still more rare. The very young child has little awareness of his body organs and functions. The case of a six year old girl who repeatedly proffered complaints about her legs, her stomach, her head, etc., in a large variety stands as an exception. Her father had been in a psychiatric hospital for three years with a diagnosis of schizophrenia. The child was simply told that her father was ill. During the prolonged absence the child identified with her father, as later shown in the course of therapy.

Learning difficulties which can be sensed and anticipated prior to the beginning of formal schooling do not properly belong in this period. Briefly, to set aside learning difficulties at this time, reference is made here to deviations from the normal pattern which occur in the child of kindergarten age when he is tested for reading readiness. The latter approach is now generally adopted, particularly in private schools. To take one example, reversal of certain consonants normally takes place initially, but almost invariably the child who clings to immature transitory reversals is found in later years to have learning difficulties owing to poor word identification.

Let us return to the three main types mentioned above: (1) the *pathology of communication* offers a complex and varied picture. Its frank manifestations are usually recognized later (at the 6 to 12 year period or even adolescence), when the symptoms are specific and obvious and they clearly interfere with social adjustment. For instance, however late the frank symptoms of *stuttering* appear, one must reach back to the oral period of development to understand its dynamics. Several studies of stuttering brought out this finding among others.[55, 56, 57, 58]

Although, as indicated above, the stuttering defect attains its full development at a later period of life, the syndrome will be described in connection with its time of onset. As often is the case with anxiety manifestations, the clinical picture is not one of specific symptoms exclusive of others. For instance, stuttering is usually accompanied by a number of neurotic manifestations mostly of the compulsive order. Stuttering itself is often, and rightly so, considered a compulsive manifestation.

Definition: There is considerable confusion regarding the nature of the speech defect as represented in the usage of the two words stuttering and stammering, which roughly correspond respectively to a tonic and clonic defect. However, it is necessary to differentiate between the two, not only because the clinical and phonetic picture differs, but so does the prognostic outlook. The speech defect with tonic manifestations (roughly corresponding to what is called stuttering) has a poorer prognosis than the defect generally recognized as stammering. The tonic manifestations are in the nature of blocks. The patient stops on certain sounds the selection of which, although not always immediately understood, is traceable to unconscious associations. For varied periods of time he cannot articulate further. He "sticks" to a letter or syllable which is related to deeply meaningful symbols. The clonic manifestations are in the nature of the repetition of speech sounds.

Both forms are often associated with involuntary movements of the face, shoulders, arms, and even the whole body. The development of the involuntary movements is progressive, roughly in the order given. There may be associated respiratory and vasomotor disturbances. Other neurotic manifestations found with the stuttering and from the same anxiety source are motor restlessness, fine motor coordination disturbances. They are of a compulsive order, such as compulsive sniffling, nailbiting, compulsive behavior, obsessional thinking, thumb sucking. Enuresis, asthma attacks, and upper respiratory infections are frequently encountered. So is asocial behavior. Hostility is marked. Severe anxiety dreams are reported, and in the course of therapy are meaningful in that they enable the patient to gain insight into early traumatizations.

Onset: In a large number of cases the onset is clearly traceable to the age of two and three and the remainder between five and eight years of age. Rarely does stuttering begin after that period, and even in such a case, it represents an exacerbation of earlier anxiety manifestations which had either been unnoticed or ignored. In the majority of cases the early symptomatic oral orientation was determined by maternal attitudes, manifested in particular in the early

218

chewing-speaking situation. Neurotic manifestations, incidentally, are often present in parental backgrounds. In connection with oral situations as referred to here, the role of left-handedness must be mentioned. It is usually in the early eating situation rather than the first school (writing) set-up that adult insistence on the change of handedness has traumatizing effects.

The following case[59] is presented because it illustrates a number of points made here about the etiology of stuttering, in particular, its origin in the oral stage of development. This child was recently seen in a social situation at the age of seventeen and a half, a charmingly feminine, freely verbal youngster who had recently entered college. Incidentally, it must be pointed out that stuttering is seldom so easily accessible to therapy, because it is seldom brought so early to the attention of the psychiatrist. As a rule, by the time a child is brought to therapy he has developed in addition to the stuttering itself a number of neurotic manifestations which make therapeutic analysis considerably more difficult.

Margot was brought to treatment at three years, three months, for a severe, predominantly tonic, speech defect of 4 months' duration, which had become progressively worse and had been handled by the family in various ways. For instance, whispering at first had helped for a few days, but the child had later stuttered while whispering. The family had also taken the habit of providing words they felt the child sought.

Family History: Paternal grandparents described as high-strung. Both are right-handed. Maternal grandfather very tense, right-handed and tended to clutter. The grandmother, a quiet person, had a normal speech. The father, 40 years old, was a prosperous manufacturer, a sensitive person with keen aesthetic drives. He was a quiet, retiring person, although he was said to like people. He was anxious, "nearly got out of his mind" when the family spent part of the previous summer near a lake, because he feared that the children might be drowned. He was right-handed. His speech was clear. He was conscious of always having been too serious. The mother, 30 years old, was right-handed. She was tense, with considerable variation in moods. She had an 18-month period of depression following the birth of the patient, during which she neglected the baby and devoted her time to the older child, "to avoid sibling rivalry." She gives as an explanation that she did not have enough physical strength to care for both children. Although the family lives in the country, the children have very little freedom in or out of the house. "It's one of those places for adults."

Personal History: The patient is the second of two children, the other child being a boy 19 months older than the patient. Pregnancy was not planned but was wanted, the home conditions being then particularly favorable. The mother suffered from nausea for 3 months and was somewhat apathetic during this pregnancy, more than with the older child. The baby was breast fed for only 10 days, feeding being interrupted because of nipple-biting. For 3 months there was difficulty with the formula, but there were no further difficulties until about 1 to 2 years, when the child developed hoarding of food, dawdling, and poor appetite. The child was left-handed but was "always changed." The mother's attitude toward the feeding radically changed when the child was 2 years old. Previous to this, because of two euthenics seminars taken at college, the mother had not interfered, but she suddenly decided that "college or no college, the child has got to eat or she will starve." The child was then a little over 2 years and the feeding became a continuous fight among mother, nurse and child. The child was considered a "discipline problem" by the mother, because during this period she messed up her food and threw it on the floor. Other habits did not offer difficulties except that the child deliberately soiled her pants to annoy her nurse, who vomited as a result. The child is a shy, inhibited little girl, who is afraid of people, especially her father and her brother. She is "an easy victim" for the brother. There was marked inconsistency in handling as regards eating and discipline. Other aspects of the child's developmental history are normal.

When first seen, the child was extremely anxious about coming to the playroom and insisted on her mother being present during the first part of the interview. Later, when the mother left, she went back several times to make sure that she was there. Her play activity consisted chiefly in cooking things for the physician to eat. There was a good deal of oral activity. She realistically chewed on toy chickens, first as children, then as food. She discovered a trumpet, the mouth-piece of which she chewed to pieces, and blew loudly numerous times into the physician's ear. As she initiated and carried out the eating activities, she said that she did not like to eat. Her speech disorder was a severe, predominantly tonic dysfunction with marked spasm of the oral and facial muscles, with occasionally two or three repetitions of a syllable. The child looked markedly anxious while the block lasted, which was, as a rule, from 5 to 20 seconds, and once the spasm was timed to have lasted 45 seconds. The physician did not remark about the speech nor did she manifest any eagerness to know what the child wanted to say. The child was compulsive about putting toys back in place, remembering where she had originally found each. She was overpolite and was overheard saying "excuse me," when she had disarranged a toy in the closet, although her back was turned to the physician. During approximately the next six play sessions there was the same predominance of oral activity, chewing the crayons, gestures of taking a toy to her mouth, then checking herself, and finally an almost constant tremor of oral muscles which was in the nature of aborted chewing motions. Other oral components were seen in the play fantasy, when she said that the girl doll was naughty. "She bite my finger." When she wanted to tell about the little girl who was naughty, she stuttered severely, repeating, "I—sh—I—sh" at least 15 times, some of which was whispered, and finally gave up.

The physician asked the mother to give chewing gum to the child and chewing-speaking games were initiated during the second play period. The child enjoyed these and made up numerous speech combinations which she repeated and also hummed. In the interview with the mother the following suggestions were made: relax rigidity of training; give more freedom; offer a great deal of oral activity, trumpets, whistles, lollipops, chewing gum; allow messy activities in specially arranged space; leave the speech disorder completely alone; no coercion; no help. It was suggested that the child, who was over-neatly dressed, come to the office in overalls. Gradually the child became less anxious, more self-assertive, and enjoyed making up words and play with words. After several sessions, while driving with her mother and brother, she kept the mother's attention for 15 minutes by using a language which was absolutely unintelligible to the mother. This was used not only as a play with words but also as a weapon, because her brother pleaded to know what the patient said; the mother implied that the conversation was a secret between herself and the patient. There was an indication that her dreams were connected with some aggressive activity, because in the course of play when the physician was to sleep, the latter made the statement that she had been dreaming. The child shouted at her, "That's too angry!" In answer to the inquiry as to who was angry, the child said, "Me." The patient became more and more aggressive in the play sessions and later also developed an interest in taking temperatures. There was coincident with this, some interest in feces, and she once challenged the physician about making a "B.M. on the floor," although she did not carry out the threat. Coincident with the release of anxiety and the appearance of aggressive behavior, the child's speech disorder took on a different characteristic, that is to say, it became predominantly clonic. The mother was seen at intervals and a discussion of instinctual drives and the emotional needs of children took place, with the recommendation that the child be given as much freedom and sympathetic understanding as possible for what was going to be a trying period of aggressive behavior at home. In the course of these interviews, the mother came to develop some insight into her own feeling reactions in which she expressed a preference for the older child, her rejection of the little girl, and an ambivalent attitude toward her married life which had interrupted a successful career as a buyer and the expression of other talents. She was encouraged to resume her artistic expression and found a great deal of release of tension in so doing.

Another trend which was manifested in the child's play was a fantasy of being a boy as big as her brother. She identified herself closely with him and while ill with a cold she cut her hair, explaining later to the physician that she wanted to be a boy, and also that she was angry because her mother would not let her come to the office on account of the cold.

The child continued noticeably more aggressive in the play sessions, usually giving the role of child to the physician, while she herself, as the mother, carried out aggressive activities in which the physician was to ingest food. She would get very angry and try to push objects into the ears and eyes of the physician, saying, "If you don't take it down this way, you take it down that way," which undoubtedly gave her an opportunity for abreaction of her own feelings. After a period of three months of intensive treatment, the child was free, easy, more aggressive toward her brother and her parents reported that the most conspicuous change at home was that the child was happy. She also eats well, she continues her chewing-speaking games, and her speech is free of stuttering.

It can be seen from this case, as would be with many others, that the mother-child relationship in the early chewing-speaking situation is of great importance (oral deprivation). That the mothers of children stutterers are anxious individuals is brought out by a number of studies. The oral orientation of the early anxiety at the critical phase of the child's speech development is also typical. Even the forceful change in handedness has an affective component, since it is first exerted in the eating-speaking configuration. Anxiety, always present in cases of stuttering, is not viewed as a manifestation secondary to the impairment of social communication. It must be pointed out that as a secondary manifestation, it increases the severity of defect in social communication.

(2) In the area of *disturbances of social relations and behavior* almost any deviations can be found, but standing out are the *impulsions, aggressive behavior, asocial* and *antisocial* behavior. Impulsiveness is to a large extent characteristic of the young child's behavior. This is readily understood, since during this age period the child is only slowly acquiring control over his instinctual urges. However, owing to anxiety and threats to the integrity of the ego we may find impulsion of such severe intensity that the child has not even minimal control. Coincidentally and in apparent contradistinction with these impulses, there may be great passivity, over-dependence on parents, especially the mother, and, in general, an unreadiness and unwillingness to face the reality world. Indeed, some of these children at a later time show separation from reality

and may develop a frank schizophrenic illness. As already indicated, aggressive impulses in a child of preschool age are normal manifestations. Gradually, toward the end of this period direct aggression is normally sublimated and partially controlled.

The child who shows aggressive behavior and severe impulsions is more likely to come to treatment early than the child who withdraws. Impulsions are usually of an aggressive nature, from mild repeated aggressions to the impulsion to kill and destroy. They are usually outwardly directed but can also be turned inward. Some of these children have very strong urges to destroy either animate or inanimate objects. In the first case we find repeated acts of cruelty and destructiveness toward animals, in the second case severe destructiveness, fire setting, etc.

Billy, for instance, was brought to treatment at the age of eight years. He was an only child of divorced parents (parents divorced when the child was one year old), a very bright youngster (I.Q. 150). His problem centered upon the type of behavior here discussed, impulses to kill, drive to set fires (he had caused several serious fires in and out of their house). In addition, he was unable to find his place in any social group and had been rejected from several schools. The symptoms as briefly sketched here had been of at least four years' duration. He had been taken from psychiatrist to psychiatrist, from school to school, with no results for obvious reasons. He was a pawn in the hands of very disturbed parents, whose severe conflicts were being worked out through him. The boy had never had a sense of belonging and a sense of being loved by either parent because of the conflict between them. He had been left with his mother and was closely identified with her, which was an additional source of conflict. He engaged in feminine activities, but was at the same time resentful of being thwarted in his attempt toward achieving maleness. This child had been known, since the age of at least three years, to tear legs from living frogs and injure pet animals. A number of accidents which had happened to occasional playmates were traced to him, though not recognized by him as his own responsibility. Subsequent developments show him in adolescence as a frank psychopathic personality, with lying, stealing, and physical aggression on others as part of his personality disturbances.

(3) A syndrome which almost invariably has its onset during this age period, although it is generally not recognized and brought to treatment at this time (generally six to twelve or even later), is the *obsessive-compulsive neurosis*. It is often said that severe neurosis in the child is rare.[60] This is questionable. While the child's defenses against anxiety may be marked by more plasticity and less rigidity and consequently be more amenable to treatment, there are, nevertheless, emotional disturbances which, for all the young years of the patient, are as difficult of approach as emotional disturbances in the adult. For instance, one needs only to consider the extreme of emotional disturbance in children, i.e., schizophrenia, to be convinced that anxiety and the defenses against it can be as personality-damaging and treatment-resistant in the child as in the adult.

This is true also of *obsessive-compulsive illness*. We are familiar with mild compulsions in the young child operating as defenses against anxiety. This refers to the young child walking over cracks or on cracks in the sidewalk, taking three steps and touching the wall, or demanding that the same story without one syllable changed be read at bed time or that the shade be halfway up and not all the way up, etc. A drive for sameness, a drive for reassurance through gesture or word, are normally exhibited by the young child. But these are not, properly speaking, compulsive acts in the neurotic sense considered here. And at this point, it may be in order to define obsessive thoughts and compulsive acts as neurotic phenomena.

The case of Nan is in point. A seven-year-old girl with an I.Q. of 130 came to treatment with a complaint that was a classical picture of the obsessive-compulsive syndrome. She had been in treatment elsewhere for three years with the same complaint, i.e., her obsessive thoughts and compulsive acts had begun at approximately three to four years of age. In her first contact she had complained primarily of night terrors, and the difficulty appeared to be one of severe anxiety. However, in the course of treatment beginning at seven years she had brought out a multiplicity of obsessive thoughts and

225

compulsive acts which had not been brought out even during the first period of treatment. This is a very general pattern, and it is remarkable indeed that children so young would so successfully block manifestations which they feel as not only alien but heavily laden with guilt. It can be said that, almost invariably, children who are brought in later years for a well-defined obsessive-compulsive neurosis have experienced thoughts and acts as described here, which they not only guarded against any intrusion but in addition took great pains to rationalize about, when inquiries were forced upon them. In the record of these children are found accounts of a variety of phobias between the ages of two and four, but the protective mechanisms are not known to the parents. These children are ready with—to the parents, though not satisfactorily to themselves—plausible explanations.

The case of a boy, Jeff, seen at eleven years, brought out these points with great conviction. Although the onset was said to have been fairly recent, the boy in the course of therapy clearly indicated that the multiplicity of obsessive thoughts and compulsive acts of great complexity from which he suffered, when first seen, went back to the age of two and three. As time passes the multiplicity and complexity of these phenomena increase to the point where it becomes impossible for the child to function in any sphere, intellectual, social, etc. He becomes immensely and in some cases even totally preoccupied with the abnormal phenomena.

The complexity of these pathological phenomena and the defenses against them even in the young child are illustrated by brief reference to the case of Jeff, previously published.[61]

He said he "must do everything in fours" (which made it difficult to hold his attention at school). This was a very involved scheme: "the thing I want to look at last, I look at first, then last, second before last" etc. This was described as his "base." The base must always be four-cornered; for instance, upon entering a room, if he looked at a point on a wall, he must immediately look for three other points. If no convenient point is available or visible, he must fall back on some part of his body, fingers, toes, eyes, etc., and visualize a base. If, in going from one corner of the base to the next, in a compulsory sequence, he overlooks one, he must start all over again. It is easy to understand how the simplest activity became fraught with insurmountable difficulties, and in particular how concentrating on any task became impossible. His previous summer's experience at camp was "ruined" by the fact that the partitions were made up of knotted pine, and the maze of knots prevented him from establishing safe "bases." Walls, with their minute surface imperfections, were preferred because "I know the walls are always going to be there. I feel safe to look at them." Furthermore, and perhaps more troublesome, is his obsessive thought regarding a long, flexible pipe-like structure issuing from his chest, in the region of the upper sternum. He knows this is only a thought, that there can be no pipe coming out of his chest. However, he must behave as if the pipe were there, and move in such a way that no one, or no object, crosses the mid-line in front of him. He adds that the reason that the pipe is "rubber-like" is to allow some leeway, and demonstrates the complex maneuvers he uses to avoid the pipe being "tangled up . . . the line has to bend . . . so I try to walk around (the other person) catch up around him, then I am straight again."

EMOTIONAL DISTURBANCES OF THE SIX TO TWELVE YEAR PERIOD

Viewed as a whole the emotional disturbances of this period can be classified under two main headings, not all inclusive: neurotic manifestations and psychotic manifestations.

There is a *continuance of emotional disturbances* earlier described, with some of them taking more specific and intensive forms. This is the case with *learning difficulties,* with the *obsessive-compulsive syndromes* (including stuttering) and the *psychosomatic manifestations. Anorexia nervosa* which usually proceeds from earlier feeding difficulties very often has its onset as a clinical picture during this age period.

Conspicuous among psychotic manifestations is *schizophrenia,* which will be described in some detail. Let us recall that more than half of all hospital beds are occupied by emotionally disturbed patients, and of these more than half are schizophrenics. The *affective psychoses* are very rare. *Charac-*

ter neurosis, which is found as a definite entity during the next age period, has its beginnings at this time.

Probably the most common emotional disturbance found in this age group goes under the description of *anxiety states* or *anxiety neuroses.* We have glimpsed earlier into the disorganizing effects of neurotic anxiety and the threat it represents to the integrity of the personality. We have also seen in what disturbed parent-child relationship the neurotic anxiety can arise.

Neurotic anxiety presents itself in a variety of configurations. We have seen it in its earliest form, the single anxiety attack generally repeated. The intermittence of the attacks does not mean lesser severity. The case of Elly illustrated this type of anxiety manifestation. Anxiety can manifest itself in a chronic almost continuous state or intermittently in the form of acute attacks. It can be so severe and the defenses against the anxiety can so completely fail that separation from reality and disintegration of the ego take place (unity of the personality now broken).

The following case illustrates this extreme of extreme anxiety without loss of contact with reality. Robert is an eleven-year-old boy, the second of four children, in a family where the mother and the older brother are in treatment for severe neurotic problems. He is brought to treatment for severe anxiety which is manifested primarily in his home. He is fairly comfortable at school, and there, in fact, does very well academically and socially. On the other hand, at home he is in a constant panic with the feeling that somebody is lurking from any point in his house to kidnap or kill him. He cannot stay alone in the house, and if the circumstances are such that he would have to, he prefers to go in the street. When at home, he doesn't let his mother out of his sight, following her everywhere and unable to be at rest even if she is on another floor. At the age of nine he entered treatment elsewhere for similar complaints.

There is a very disturbed parent-child relationship. Both parents have been severely punitive toward the patient. The father is immature, strongly tied up to his mother, who is a matriarchal domineering type. In fact, the family at the beginning of the marriage lived with paternal grandparents for

228

this reason. He tends to escape from painful realities by suddenly leaving his home, usually under the guise of lengthy business trips, but also as an avowed expression of his inability to cope with life situations. The mother has been in analysis for close to two years. She has had an emotionally deprived childhood and has made a neurotic adjustment to life situations including her marriage. Until her analysis started, the husband-wife relationship was definitely a sado-masochistic one. She has begun to assert herself and stand up against her husband's infantile and arbitrary demands. Hers has been a continuous story of disorganizing anxiety. She brings out, for instance, that she interrupted her training in a profession because of her fear of certain students. She was then in her early twenties. A great deal of underlying aggressiveness and hostility are brought forth in the course of her therapy, and her underlying drive to manage is now explicit.

Birth conditions were difficult and the child was partly cyanotic. This is a point worthy of note in the light of the previously mentioned observations on the predisposition to anxiety. The early family background, with a very insecure and anxious mother and an overpowering and immature father, was not any more favorable. It is significant that the mother remembers little about the early development, having put the first two children in the hands of a nurse. That there was oral deprivation is clearly indicated by the history and the fact that he still sucks on his fingers when under stress. There was a period when the finger sucking was so severe as to interfere with functioning, social relationships, schooling, etc. He has had sleeping difficulties throughout, from the age of approximately two years, about the time when his next sibling was born. Shortly after this, he had a tonsillectomy, which was traumatic owing to the already present anxiety. Life in Robert's home is very difficult, because at eleven years his demands are those of an infant who cannot be at any moment left alone.

Robert is an attractive boy of very superior intelligence who is obviously under great tension as he sits on the edge of his chair in the playroom. Nevertheless, he tells fairly freely of his varied anxieties. An intelligent boy, he is fully aware that it is irrational to think that a witch or a giant would be about to destroy him. Nevertheless, he is constantly preoccupied with these thoughts. He lives with a sense of impending danger and threat of total destruction. He is afraid of getting hurt, afraid of dying. He cannot go from one floor to the next in his house unless at least one of his siblings comes along. He prefers his mother to accompany him. When alone, he hears loud noises, the source of which he cannot always trace. These noises, however, are not in the nature of auditory hallucinations. His mother, he feels, is an overpowering manager, and he had great anxiety about his father, who in a jolly way is a back slapper. He has come to fear the slightest touch from his father. "He pinches me in a friendly manner. Sometimes I feel he is a robber and I get scared."

There is evidence of confusion in the male-female identification, verbally as well as projected in drawings. During a subsequent interview he revealed that he had thought of the psychiatrist as a witch who was in command of giants ready to kill him. The giants he visualized hiding in the cupboards of the playroom. He often feels that "a crazy man is waiting for me to kill me." Misinterpretation of external stimuli is part of the picture, and a radio giving out what sounded definitely like a soap opera was interpreted by him as the radio of a police station with which the office would be connected. Some of the internal experiences reported by this boy could easily be viewed as psychotic manifestations, were it not that the boy himself insists on his awareness of the irrationality of these experiences. Against the overwhelming anxiety, defenses are to a large extent ineffectual, and there can be no question that it is a matter of time before a complete break with reality takes place, unless therapy is instituted and effectual. Even then, it must be kept in mind that the picture is very close to ego disintegration and forecasts the appearance of psychotic manifestations. The break with reality seems imminent, though a diagnosis of schizophrenia cannot be made at this time.

Schizophrenia: Of the psychotic illnesses found in children schizophrenia, which was some twenty years ago seldom reported or recognized, has now become the most prominent. Even reckoning with the present tendency to over-diagnose schizophrenic illness in childhood, the fact remains that there has been an increase in this illness, which is primarily an ego disease. The increasing trend is to be kept in mind when considering ego development within the family. One cannot escape bringing together two facts: the increase of ego disease in the child, on the one hand, and on the other, the weakening of the family structure with the correlated increase in disturbances of parent-child relationships.

This is not the place for a lengthy history of the disease, and only a few meaningful sequences are here given. While the literature on childhood schizophrenia has been mounting rapidly, it is only in recent years that this illness has been associated with childhood. To give the reader an idea of this increase we need only mention a bibliography of childhood schizophrenia published in 1956.[62] The bibliography lists 584 articles and/or books on the subject, "as reported in the English language through 1954."

Bender, reporting in 1955 on twenty years of research on schizophrenic children, indicates that 850 schizophrenic children aged 2 to 12 (i.e., 8% of the total 7,000) were admitted during the period of 1934-1954 to the children's service of the Bellevue Psychiatric Division.[63]

In the United States probably the first significant definition as applied to childhood was given by Potter in 1933, when he reported on six cases of childhood schizophrenia (age on admission: 4, 6, 10, 11, 11, 12).[64] Between 1932 and 1935 two Russian psychiatrists, Ssucharewa[65] and Grebelskaja-Albatz, 66 published extensive reports on a large number of cases of child schizophrenia of various types which they had observed. The first author reported on 107 children from 7 to 17 years, the second on 22 cases from 3½ to 8 years. Lauretta Bender in 1937 included the case of a schizophrenic child in a study of behavior problems in the children of psychotic and criminal parents.[67] The patient was an eleven-year-old girl with an I.Q. of 87 who was described as "a remarkable case of paranoid schizophrenia." That childhood schizophrenia was considered rare is clearly brought out in Bender's discussion of hereditary influences and relationships between psychoses of parents and emotional disturbances in their children. "The evidence points to the fact that schizophrenia in a parent may predispose to neurotic traits in other members of the family and the social or mental maladjustment to some

231

extent in children, but not necessarily to schizophrenia or schizoid features. Of the offspring of schizophrenic parents, 25% are reported to be psychotic, and of these none developed the psychosis in childhood." The writer presented in 1937 at the First International Congress of Child Psychiatry a series of 29 schizophrenic children admitted at New York State Psychiatric Institute from 1930 to 1937 and who had been followed for from one and a half to six years. Nine children (8 boys, 1 girl) were under seven years of age, and the remaining twenty (15 boys, 5 girls) were seven to thirteen years of age at admission.

The diagnostic criteria in that early stage of recognition of the disease in children were adapted from the adult illness, as shown by the criteria formulated by Potter.[68] He lists them as follows:

1. A generalized retraction of interests from the environment.
2. Dereistic thinking, feeling, acting.
3. Disturbances of thought, manifested through blocking, symbolization, condensation, perseveration, incoherence, and diminution, sometimes to the extent of mutism.
4. Defect in emotional rapport.
5. Diminution, rigidity and distortion of affect.
6. Alterations of behavior with either an increase of motility, leading to incessant activity, or a diminution of motility, leading to complete immobility or bizarre behavior with a tendency to perseveration or stereotypy.

A more recent definition offered by Bender covers so many areas of dysfunction as to permit the inclusion of cases which do not correspond to schizophrenic illness as earlier defined in the adult. Organicity, for instance, is necessarily included in this definition, although schizophrenic illness as defined by Bleuler precludes organicity. Bender defined schizophrenia in children as:

A clinical entity, occurring in childhood before the age of eleven years, which reveals pathology in behavior at every level and in every area of integration or patterning within the functioning of the central nervous system, be it vegetative, motor, perceptual, intellectual, emotional, or social.

Furthermore, this behavior pathology disturbs the pattern of every functioning field in a characteristic way. The pathology cannot therefore be thought of as local in the architecture of the central nervous system, but rather as striking at the substratum of integrative functioning or biologically patterned behavior.[69]

A definition by the writer which seems to comply with the diagnostic requirements of the disease entity of schizophrenia as originally described in adults and allowing for developmental differences in children is given as follows. "A disease process in which the loss of affective contact with reality is coincident with or determined by the appearance of autistic thinking and accompanied by specific phenomena of regression and dissociation."[70]

Another formulation, Mahler's, has attempted to differentiate between autistic and symbiotic types of schizophrenic illness in children.[71] Although clinically the differentiation is not as clear as formulated, it deserves further investigation. Others, such as Rank, have included schizophrenia under large groups of psychoses, their common denominator being atypicality.[72] More recently the stress on deviated ego functions in schizophrenic illness has been noted by Beres.[73]

The definitions advanced above for schizophrenia are avowedly descriptive and do not concern themselves with the dynamics of the illness.

Schizophrenia considered dynamically is essentially a disease of the ego, a point on which most authors agree. Let us recall that in 1924 Freud, in "The Loss of Reality in Neurosis and Psychosis," formulated that the alienation of the ego was the central disturbance in the psychoses of adolescence and adulthood. In 1938 Schilder in "The Image Appearance of the Human Body" formulated a concept of the body image, a psychic projection or representation of the body self. He found this to be the initial and central core of ego development. Through the body image representation the separation of the infant from the mother is gradually achieved. This is the first awareness of external reality. The mother is at first and for a matter of months the only external reality of the infant, who originally lives in both physiological and affective

233

symbiosis with her. Ribble, among others, has concurred with this concept.

These observations are of prime importance in relation to the pathology of childhood schizophrenia as an ego disease. Its origins are in the pregenital phase of psycho-sexual development. This assertion is supported by the predominance in the child schizophrenic of omnipotence fantasies, oral and anal aggressive fantasies, and an enormous anxiety over identity of self (man or animal, male or female).

The symptoms of schizophrenia vary in relation to chronological age and psycho-sexual development. Several outstanding and well-known observations must be emphasized here. Reality-testing is a function of the ego. As we have seen, ego differentiation from external reality is reflected in the evolution of language forms. The "I—not-I," for instance, an awareness of which the child has achieved in terms of the body at the end of the first year, is reached in terms of affectivity toward the end of the third year. At this time the normal child of average intelligence uses the first person when referring to himself. The schizophrenic child, however, talks about himself in the third person, singular or plural, considerably later than this age. In fact, adolescent and adult schizophrenics may continue to do so.

With the young child in the pre-language phase, verbal expressions cannot be relied on as an index of inner conflict. Behavior patterns and emotional manifestations must be the basis for clinical observation.

It is often difficult to ascertain the content of delusional experiences in the young child, even when it is obvious that he reacts to visual and auditory hallucinations. The child frequently identifies with animals, projecting upon them his own instinctual impulses, using these animals both as destroyers and as victims. The range of animals is wide, but there is a predominance of the devouring type. The case of a four-year-old schizophrenic boy previously reported[74] should be mentioned here. Identifying with a dog while ill at the beginning of therapy, he would snarl by reverting to a primitive muscular pattern.

The schizophrenic child lives in an inner reality which has little reference to the external reality world. From the age of seven on hallucinations in all sensory spheres are common. The younger the child, the simpler, less organized, and more primitive are these hallucinations. From the age of ten or eleven the patterns are very similar to those of the adult.

The inner reality of the schizophrenic child represents an attempt to escape from the anxiety aroused by the conflict between instinctual drives and repressive forces issuing from the external reality world, as originally extended from parents. The escape does not resolve the anxiety, and it is obvious to the observer that the child lives in a state of continuous, intense anxiety. If the anxiety of the neurotic is measured in volts, that of the schizophrenic is measured in millions of volts, says John Rosen, who has had considerable experience with this. This anxiety often appears in the form of acute panics, often at first misinterpreted as temper tantrums.

Dissociative phenomena are also a reflection of the child's effort at separating the self from the external reality world. This can be seen in the monotonous, mechanical quality of the voice, in the motor stereotypes, in the bizarre motor patterns, and in the language patterns.

One of the early manifestations of schizophrenic illness, one most frequently found and which can be considered a pathognomic sign of disturbance in ego development in these children (especially in early infantile autism) is dissociation between language as a sign and language as a function. The child thus has the capacity to acquire and use words mechanically, some of them very difficult words representing complex concepts. But he has only a meager vocabulary to express his own needs in terms of emotional relationships. Mutism and/or neologisms may also be present. The frequent addiction of these children to music is of the same abstract, dissociative order. Kanner was among the first to call attention to the significance of music to the schizophrenic child.

Dissociation is also seen in the affective sphere. There may be withdrawal or distortion of affect. A mother reports of her son. "He tells a story with an expression that would apply to another story." The child may have an interest in topics quite out of the interest range for his age group—astronomy, highly intellectual technicalities, the knowledge of the dynamics of automobiles and machinery, higher mathematics, etc.

—all inappropriate concerns for any child from five to ten years of age.

To the point of having no identity of his own, the child identifies closely with personages remote in time and space (ancient times, Civil War, etc.) and with animals.

There is evidence in the schizophrenic child of the contingency and co-existence of considerably varied levels of maturity. Primitive fantasies and regressive behavior (soiling, wolfing food, etc.) may exist side by side with reasoning at a high intellectual level. The failure of ego organization is evident here, and ego fragmentation is a conspicuous feature. The child has failed to develop as one, as a differentiated individual, in his rejection of the reality world.

The parents of these children have quite distinctive characteristics. Kanner has commented on the intellectual and remote character of their personalities.

A few words should be said about the fluidity of the body stressed by Bender and her followers. There are as many children with rigid, automatic motor attitudes as children characterized by this body fluidity. Both extremes are seen.

Motor behavior toward objects is of the same order. The child may cling as if he were part of another in symbiosis, but not as if he regarded the person as a human being. Or, on the other extreme, he may use the lap of parent or therapist as nothing more than a seat, an inanimate object. He may "walk through" a person as if that person did not exist. It is up to the other person to clear the space. Both types of behavior show an evident loss of awareness of external reality. Similarly, there may be a lack of sensitivity to pain.

Psychotherapy is based on the concept that schizophrenic illness represents an attempt at denying and fleeing from reality in order to resolve overwhelming anxiety. By all means at his disposal the therapist must break into the autistic world of the child. This presents great difficulties, since that autistic world is restricted and often, on first contact, unintelligible. This is particularly true of early infantile autism. One is impressed by the determination of the child not to communicate, a determination so intense that he may punish himself severely, biting, hitting his head against a wall, etc., when

236

arises the first desire and attempt to communicate in conflict with the earlier determination not to. Some of these children show great anxiety when addressed, putting their fingers in their ears, whispering to themselves, repeating words singsong, rocking, etc.

A Case:[75] Mary, twelve and a half years old at the time of writing, was first seen at nine and a quarter years of age. She is the oldest of three children (two younger brothers) in a family of middle-class social and economic status. She had been treated for two previous periods elsewhere, beginning at the age of five and a half. There was no question that the child was schizophrenic, a diagnosis in which everyone concurred.

She was a very odd-looking child, oldish, with poor contact and almost incoherent when first seen. Overactive, she wandered about the playroom, paying no attention to the examiner, talking to herself, in loud, incoherent words with an unnatural voice. The emotional tone is inappropriate: either expressionless, or laughing as she tells gruesome fantasies. With all the incoherence, some fragments of speech can be projected in a frame of reference belonging to an early situation.

Going into the family background and the early years throws a light on the meaning of these fragments.

The father, in his late thirties, the second of two boys who said of his brother still living, "I had a brother"—is a professional man who doesn't mingle easily, feels lonesome and was for two years actually isolated from his family because of pulmonary tuberculosis, now arrested. In addition, he was in the Armed Forces from the time of the child's birth to 17 months, during which period the mother lived with her parents, and the child became close to her grandfather, calling him Daddy.

The mother, also in her late thirties, is the older of two girls and is still very close to her family; a vigorous and domineering woman who described herself in the following terms: "I am a driving woman. I have compulsive cleanliness, moodiness, and I am a little paranoid." She was for several years an occupational therapist in a state institution for mental diseases, and made the diagnosis of schizophrenia on her child —correctly—before the first period of treatment.

With regard to development, birth was normal and so was the infant's early emotional response. Thumb-sucking has persisted to date, and elimination training seems to have been free of tension. She was reared in the home of maternal grandparents while the mother worked. She called her grandfather "Daddy" and at 17 months was told for the first time that her daddy was coming home. The grandfather was "extremely jealous" of the father, in spite of which both parents insist that the child "took right away to her father because of his uniform buttons." However, it is noted that the child, who had started to talk early, stopped at 18 months. Furthermore, in the course of treatment, the child has frequently referred to her confusion over these two fathers, and many fantasies involve grandfather as alternately dead and alive. At three and a half, after her first brother was born, she actively lived the fantasy of two imaginary companions, one good little boy, and one bad, each one with his own name. At about 6 years she fused the two under the bad boy's name. When the brother was one year old, she asked for an axe to "chop his head." She was 7 when her maternal grandfather died. (In therapeutic sessions, she has given the time as 3½, i.e., when her brother was born.) The grandfather had died suddenly, following a chest operation for carcinoma of the lungs, and the child expressed then, and still does, crucifixion fantasies involving her grandfather as "Daddy," herself, and, less frequently, other members of her family and people outside of her family. She would not go to school without a large doll which occupied a desk next to hers, and with whom she engaged in long, whispered conversations.

It was further established in the course of therapy that the grandfather had died while she had a tonsillectomy at the same hospital. She insisted she had seen her grandfather's body wheeled on a stretcher past her open door. While she actually had been at the hospital as a patient when her grandfather died, she had not seen him then; neither could she have seen his body go past her room, since she was in a different wing. The experience thus reported was unquestionably hallucinatory.

She showed intense preoccupation with death, graves, cemeteries. A grave "game" in particular showed "everybody dead . . . I am dead . . . if Grandpa doesn't behave in his grave, he'll be dead too"—world-destruction fantasies, omnipotence fantasies ("everything is destroyed except me . . . I'm too smart . . . I'm a God"). Her own death and fantasies of rebirth were also acted out. Identified with her grandfather, she was crucified with her "chest cut open."

Foremost, the purpose of therapy is to establish contact. To this effect, the meaning of apparently incoherent fragments is unravelled, the symbolism of neologisms, distorted and autistic experiences brought to consciousness. Once contact is established and some transference developed, therapy is no different than that of the severe neurotic.

At this time Mary is functioning in a limited way, able to progress in school with a one-year lag, and while still somewhat odd in behavior and verbal symbolism, she is capable of attending to her tasks in reality situations, has a few friends, and enters new situations with moderate ease.

One cannot speak of complete recovery except in those few cases where the personality is fairly intact and ego development before an acute episode was reasonably good. When the development of the illness has been insidious and ego development inadequate, the prognosis is poor.

EMOTIONAL DISTURBANCES OF THE TWELVE TO EIGHTEEN YEAR PERIOD

Neuroses and psychoses as found in the previous age group are, of course, found here, with further intensification and clearer delineation of types. The *affective psychoses* (manic-depressive illness) which are so rarely noted in the previous age group increase somewhat in frequency—although not to the degree of that found in the adult, nor is the clinical picture so frank an entity. With the adolescent there is often an admixture of symptoms belonging to schizophrenic illness. Whether the illness without therapy will evolve toward manic-depressive or schizophrenic illness is not as a rule definable during this period.

Prior to this age group one cannot speak of *character neurosis*. The plasticity and flexibility of the child's character prior to adolescence preclude such a development. Franz Alexander was probably the first to formulate the concept of character neurosis, making careful study of the dynamics involved.[76] Reaction-formation as a defense against instinctual impulses (sadistic, for instance) results from the failure of their sublimation. The reaction-formation in a case discussed led to excessive drive for knowledge, becoming part of the personality as such. There is a restriction of interest in the social sphere and the overintellectualization substitutes for emotional interchanges. Character neurosis is actually crystallized toward the end of this period, i.e., close to adulthood. Much has been written on the subject since Alexander, for the most part dealing with adults.

Two phases of emotional disturbances during this period deserve special consideration because of their importance during this age period: *juvenile delinquency* and *sexual problems.*

Juvenile delinquency has in recent years become a social problem of such magnitude that special committees for the study of all its varied aspects have been formed. Much time has been expended on these investigations which have involved authorities in the fields of psychiatry, sociology, and psychology. Some of their findings have been incorporated in Hendrickson's inclusive report, *Youth in Danger.*[77]

That juvenile delinquency should be more marked during the adolescent period and should be now on the increase can be understood in terms of the breaking down of the family. The latter can take place under the impact of various factors, and these are presented at length in Hendrickson's report. Let us recall that adolescence is normally a period of emancipation from parental authority, and also that internal pressures are increased owing to developments which are specific to this age period and which have been discussed earlier. Some index of the magnitude of this problem is found in the statistical figures. Says Hendrickson, "more than one million youngsters in America this year will find their way into trouble by 1960. Unless we do something about it the figures will probably mount to 1,700,000." Although, even in the face of such figures, his point of view is far from being pessimistic, the statistics given are tale-telling. He points out, for instance, that the number of juvenile delinquents "is only about 1/18th of the population between ten and seventeen years of age." And only one third of this total, some 435,000 or less "are involved in antisocial activities for which they are brought to court. Obviously, were the figures concentrated in the upper age span of this group their meaning in terms of percentage of the population would be altered."

Sociological factors are carefully considered, especially the influence of slums and of low socio-economic status. For instance, a study was made of a group of families living in a Washington, D.C., slum. Two hundred and twenty-two people lived in a block of forty houses. Half of them were children. A sampling of half of this total group was made. Fifty-two children were thus included, half of them six years of age or under. Only eight of these children lived with both father and mother; twenty-eight lived with their mother; four lived with their grandmother. Sixteen of these children were readily reported by mother or grandmother to have been born out of wedlock. As seen here, the stress is on sociological factors. But even as sociological factors are considered, one cannot escape the glaring fact of family breakdown, and in particular the emotional deprivation from the removal of one or both parents, the father being the conspicuous absentee.

The instability of war years is advanced as a factor in the increase of juvenile delinquency. Considering only antisocial acts so severe as to be brought to the attention of the courts, Hendrickson's report brings out sharp increases in delinquency during war years, with a low ebb before the Second World War.

In 1940, approximately 235,000 children in the United States were coming to the attention of the courts for delinquent behavior. During World War II, this nearly doubled, with 400,000 being brought into juvenile courts in both 1943 and 1945. After World War II delinquency decreased until, in 1948, there were again fewer than 300,000 youth in serious trouble.

Again, in interpreting the curve of rise and fall of figures in its relation to the state of war two facts must be recalled: the breaking apart of the family and the absence of the father, with all its repercussions on personality development as previously discussed. In addition, one must not lose sight of the fact that the figures given in this report include only what one might call "official" juvenile delinquency. There is a gamut of antisocial acts which are never brought to court, as can be recalled from illustrations given earlier.

The role of the mother, especially as it is currently affected by social conditions, also has a bearing on the subject. Figures are given for 1953 about the total number of children under eighteen years of age in the United States (52,400,000), the total number of mothers (5.3 million) and the proportion in the latter group of mothers with children under eighteen years of age (5.2 million). However, it is difficult to give an adequate evaluation of the maternal factor, since we do not know, for instance, how many of these children are under six years of age. We must rely on individual observations, quoted at intervals, to assess the role of the mother.

The well-known studies of the Gluecks[78] are included in the report, together with extensive interviews of the authors. Let it be recalled that the Gluecks studied five hundred delinquent boys in comparison with five hundred non-delinquent boys aged ten to seventeen, matching them on the basis of physical, intellectual, emotional, and, as far as possible, economic factors. The parents of the delinquent children showed a marked degree of delinquency themselves—66% of the fathers had criminal records and 50% of the mothers had records of crime or delinquency. These figures are considerably above those applying to non-delinquents. Evidence of instability was shown in the prevalence of alcoholism among the parents, and the inadequacy and helplessness of the parents were brought out in their ready tendency to turn to agencies in their arbitration of internal domestic problems. Again, the adequacy and self-reliance of families of the non-delinquent group is in contrast with the other group.

One is impressed with the fact that in eight out of ten of the families of delinquents the family lacked unity and emotional warmth, and there was a prevalence of broken homes. Of particular interest is the fact that in eight out of ten of the broken homes the break had occurred when the boys were under ten years of age. The father-son, mother-son relationships were disturbed, with hostility or indifference on the part of the parent a conspicuous factor.

Drug addiction, generally included in delinquency figures, has been on the increase, and a need created for the building of hospitals, the special purpose of which is therapy for drug addiction in adolescence.

Sexual problems are another aspect of juvenile delinquency. We have seen that adolescence is a period where the whole sexual-emotional balance is disturbed, in part on a physiological basis. Working with adolescents in the capacity of psychiatrist, educator, group leader, etc., one readily becomes acquainted with the sexual conflicts encountered in this age group. Statistics here prove of little help, since many degrees of sexual delinquency escape statistical evaluation.

The increase in the number of babies born out of wedlock cannot but be of significance. Since 1952 it is impossible to get at these figures, since thirty-three states are no longer differentiating between legitimacy and illegitimacy on birth certificates. The last reliable census was in 1952. The total number of illegitimate babies—which was 87,000 in 1938—jumped to 150,300 in 1952. These figures were collated in relation to research on adoption.[79]

Compulsive behavior is the basis for many instances of *sexual promiscuousness.* The adolescent boy or girl is seeking love, which he has not received, in a form which cannot bring love to him. Over and over, he repeats the experience with the drive to reach this goal—to receive love, unable ever to grasp that love cannot be given to him in this way. These adolescents generally have a background of early parental love deprivation or distortion—mainly maternal.

The opposite is also found, i.e., sexual inhibitions, when the search for sexual satisfaction brings anxiety and guilt. The guilt is related to the sense of taboo acquired during early years, traceable again to parental attitudes. Both the sexual conflict between parents and early repressive attitudes of parents contribute to this development. Obsessive fear of venereal diseases is of this order, or it can be part of a compulsive personality.

A comment must be made about emotional disturbances

which apply to all age groups, i.e., emotional disturbances associated with *physical illness* or *physical handicap*. Much has been written about emotional disturbances found in the cardiac, physically handicapped, poliomyelitis-affected child, etc. There is a common basis for all. The threat to the body integrity represents a source of intense anxiety for the sufferer himself. But, in addition, it determines parental attitudes which come into play: a mother may be overly anxious about a cardiac condition in her child, immobilize him more than is necessary, interfere with his natural aggressive impulses, and foster emotional development in a milieu of intense anxiety.

To sum up, throughout the picture built around the emotionally disturbed child, the stress has been on the early years. This stems from a profound conviction: the early years of a child in his family are all-meaningful for his emotional development. Were it possible to conceive (avowedly a Utopian view) of families so warm and so well-integrated, as to give the maximum security, the maximum assurance of normal emotional growth to the child, it would also be possible to conceive that emotional disturbances in the child would be at a minimum.

Part Five

REFLECTIONS ON THE FAMILY

DIRECT EXPERIENCE AND SUBSTITUTES

What, today, has become of the mother in America? Amid the abundance of material on child training, with the emphasis on physical and psychological health for the young, with such organizations as the Parent-Teachers Association, why is it that children must grow up without the emotional strength which a mother—and a mother alone—can provide? This is the age of the vitamin pill, of the scientifically prepared formula, the age in which, in addition and as never before, we worship childhood and youth. In one respect, however, women today are almost consistently lacking; that is in the one essential for their children—love.

It is pointless to "blame" the mother. History has taken its toll on her. Woman's position in society has been drastically altered in the last thirty years. Once happy to be a home-maker, she has been encouraged to turn away from "drudgery" and to realize her potential to do a man's work and enjoy a man's freedom (or is a man's freedom also a myth?).

The family grows smaller and smaller. No longer do parents, grandparents, and children live together. One is unlikely to be able to turn to a sister next door for company or help. When she marries, a girl leaves her home, not to enter her husband's family (in our times not the happy solution it may have been in tribal life), but to start off alone with him. Together they will have to be all things to each other and to their children. The stress upon them is not lightened, as it was in former times, by the presence of other adults. And it is usually the mother who must bear the greater pressure of responsibility by herself, for she is naturally the focal point of family life.

The almost frantic attempts to provide children with the material benefits of our age seems to indicate that mothers are trying to compensate for their inability to give fully of their love. It is a relief, they find, to administer pills, to keep in touch with the child's teacher, to see that the girl has dancing lessons and braces on her teeth. Such attention, though of great value, cannot provide a child with the emotional security which a mother should offer. *Instinctive motherliness is being smothered in the material wealth of modern life.*

Civilization cannot rob the woman of the basic instinct to protect her young from danger. On a small scale this is evident in the irate mother who rushes to the defense of her child when criticism falls his way. Few mothers have the opportunity to show this devotion in scenes of greater danger, but there is no reason to doubt that their instincts would serve them then as well. The mother cat protects her litter from the dog; the lioness guards her cubs in the face of the hunter's gun; so would a mother risk her own life to save her child from the wheels of a car.

This type of giving still comes by instinct. But the small demands of the child are not so easy to meet. They seem to leave the mother helpless. When the child needs her attention, her time is already full. She rushes her little girl in and out of the tub, absentmindedly listening to her chatter, hurries her through dinner with a few words urging the child to eat, and sees her into bed, relieved to finally have a moment to herself. The day is over and it seems to have been devoted to chores. Without knowing it, the mother has sacrificed her time and pleasure unnecessarily. She has lost the opportunity to enjoy her child. The moments she might have had talking with him, going over the events of the day, hearing about new friends, new games, small troubles, have been lost in the rush to get her child fed and bundled into bed. These moments should not be hurried ones; they should provide the time for mother and child to get to know each other. They can only be such, when a woman forgets about being a dutiful mother with rigid inexorable standards and becomes a loving one.

No time past has seen her so diligent to learn the best and most up-to-date formulas for child care. A wealth of conflicting information pours daily from radio, television, and magazine. Advice is offered in bewildering quantity. What the mother really needs, unfortunately, cannot be taught. Were she to close her ears momentarily to the popular hucksters of opinion, she might be able to heed her own feelings. Where her intellect has failed they would guide her to her own happiness and the happiness of her children. The trend to *learn motherhood* may be a sham, and even a danger. By approaching her child intellectually the mother may create a gulf which will become increasingly difficult for them to cross.

Mothers do not only fail their children in misguided attempts at understanding them. Some have little interest even in book knowledge. Their children are at best showpieces. When they are not dressed up for company, they are considered a nuisance. In this respect we are not as far from the Victorian era as we may think.

In many cases mothers have followed the dictates of fashion and the pressures of conformism. In planning for a family they have probably entertained mental pictures of themselves as mothers: the smartly dressed young woman ready for a party, with her two children waving good-by. Shining faces, they obligingly vanish when no longer needed to complete the picture.

We have all seen some small girl solicitously putting her doll to bed when she has tired of playing with it. Or she may have simply dropped it on the floor, when something more interesting caught her attention. Many a mother is still this little girl. Her children are playthings, and she claims the right to play when her mood dictates, and only when her mood dictates. She may enjoy cuddling, feeding, and bathing her baby. But when the baby refuses to eat, when he cries in his crib, then the game is disrupted. The mother finds herself trapped. Resentment overcomes her, if she does not have the opportunity to hand her charge over to maid or nurse.

In her immaturity frustration comes as a dreadful blow. At one moment her children will suffer her rages; at the next

249

the confusion of the indulgence she has shown them in answer to her feelings of guilt. They have been deprived of a mother's love, and she in turn has been deprived of the joy of their very being. Inevitably her marriage must suffer, for the brunt of her temper will also fall on her husband. He will find that he actually has, not a mature wife, but a frustrated child on his hands.

From just such families come many mothers and children to the psychiatrist's office. Many a family of this type finally breaks down, either officially by legal divorce, or perhaps more destructively, by emotional divorce. And then the way is readied for another generation of emotionally disturbed people.

It was only thirty years ago or so that women achieved their goal, emancipation. Then was scarcely the time for them to brood over its far-reaching consequences. But now we must be concerned, for women are paying a heavy price for the victory of the previous generation.

The fight has subsided. Woman no longer demand so firmly the right to do the work that was once considered exclusively man's. In a broad measure they have this right. For over a generation their numbers in the upper levels of business and the professions have shown little fluctuation, despite increasing opportunities for women to enter man's many fields. Take medical schools, for instance. The number of women admitted there varies from ten to fifteen percent, not because the number of women accepted for training is restricted, but rather that the woman-man proportion of applications is of that order.

According to Parsons, unmarried women make up the large majority of working women today.[1] Those who marry are not long in leaving their offices and returning home. Women who follow careers are usually unmarried, and those who combine marriage and a career are surprisingly low in number. Those who do work are usually of the middle class, and they fill jobs which few men have shown a leaning for, such as typists, stenographers, and nurses.

What would the militant suffragettes of the past say of today's generation of young women who, offered every opportunity for a profession, turn down such opportunity in favor of devoting themselves full-time to home and family? Now, it is no longer their own inclination that leads women out of the home. It is most often financial necessity or war-time shortage of workers.

Women left their homes to satisfy their need to compete with men on a man's level. In gaining their freedom they unwittingly sacrificed deeper values of which they are only now becoming aware. And, aware of their loss, they are returning home, perhaps in an unconscious desire to regain their womanliness. Let it be understood that this is not a plea for a return to the relegation of women in the home. However, the need for a re-examination of the issues involved is evident. This can be done, not at the periphery, but at the core.

The job of a part-time career woman, part-time mother is too heavy for the majority of women. So many little things in the schedule of home and office go awry. What happens, for instance, when a mother is unavoidably held late at the office and her part-time maid has to go home? Her little girl, only three years old, cannot fend for herself for that hour or so, whether she was left home with a baby-sitter or waiting to be picked up at the nursery. In little ways a woman's day can become chaotic and anxiety ridden.

The difficulty is a twofold one. The physical strain is wearing, but the emotional strain on the family is even greater. A mother has very little time to enjoy her children when she must rush off each day to a job. Her children will come home to a maid, or to an empty house. When an important school event comes up, the second grade play, for instance, mother won't be able to get away in the morning to attend. Her husband suffers too. In some instances, even before he leaves in the morning his wife will be off, and when he returns home, she is not yet there. In the confusion of such an arrangement the gradual growth and maturing of the family together becomes an insoluble puzzle.

Realizing this, women are no longer sure that they want to work away from home. They have decided to return. It is their own choice. But that choice is still made with some regrets and negative overtones which tend to weigh them down. When they decided to seek careers, it was with a dissatisfaction over their roles as housekeepers. That dissatisfaction remains.

There is an undercurrent of conflict and it runs deep. In order to understand it we must consider more general trends in today's world. Society in our century is almost obsessed with individualism, while at the same time pressing on the individual the great need to conform. Women are discontented over their routine work in the house. They feel robbed of independence. The creativity that lies in the daily tasks of home and family escapes them.

How well are girls today emotionally prepared for adulthood? Inescapably, children have their earliest introduction to life around them in the home. Through their mother they first have contact with the outer world. Early, the girl has a chance to identify with her mother in womanly ways. From her example she should be able to learn simple household tasks. She may enjoy cooking her own sticky fudge concoctions while her mother works in the kitchen. This semi-play sharing of her mother's work should help her in her later role as a full-fledged housewife.

But all too few mothers can set themselves as examples of happy homemakers. A mother today usually passes on to her little girl not her enjoyment of cooking and caring for her family, but her resentment of these tasks. She hurries through her chores in the kitchen, pushing her small daughter off to go play outside. Nowadays it is no longer pressing a dime for the corner movies, but offering a seat before the T.V. set. Despite frozen foods, pressure cookers, and the automatically timed oven, housework remains a burden. Her daughter, seeing her mother's dissatisfaction, can hardly be expected to grow up in happy anticipation of caring for a home of her own. On the eve of wedding plans anticipation is poor preparation and at best figures as a delayed reaction.

The need for women who can manage a home has been recognized by many universities. To solve the problem they have added home economics courses to their curriculum. At Cornell, for instance, girls work in experimental homes where they are supervised in running a house. They plan meals, learn to shop efficiently, and for one week each girl is entrusted with the complete care of a baby.

This training is fine as far as it goes. But it is one-sided. Intellectually it suffices. But it cannot build in a girl an emotional acceptance of housework. It cannot substitute for a childhood spent with a mother who exudes her enjoyment in caring for her family. This enjoyment cannot be taught in a university. And enjoyment alone can turn housework from drudgery to satisfying creative work.

When a girl grows up hearing her mother's constant complaints about being tied down to her home, that girl, both consciously and unconsciously, will grow to resent any demands housework might make upon her. She will not feel satisfaction in helping her mother, or, later, in caring for her own family.

Many such girls enter the home economics courses offered by universities. They come totally unprepared. Some have never cooked a meal. They do not expect to enjoy their work, but to master it.

It is something of a contradiction that mothers, feeling as they do about housework, expect their daughters to offer help around the home. When they complain about their daughters' indifference to household tasks, they fail to realize that they have contributed to this indifference.

Advertising plays a large part in giving housework the unpleasant connotations it has today. Magazines offer one picture after another of dream kitchens where dinner does all but prepare itself. It comes from the freezer to the table as if by magic. The housewife will soon be obsolete, if mechanization proceeds at its present rate. Garbage melts away in the drain. Dishes create no problem with the automatic dish washer. Outside of the kitchen, the vacuum cleaner offers a variety of services, from its traditional function of removing dust to its most recent feats which include painting a wall. Promoters, of course, know of the vulnerability and intellectual lethargy of their public.

Advertisements promise us all these things. But even with the most up-to-date equipment, the home is not yet the machine-made paradise advertisers would have us believe. Some women are blissfully unaware of this discrepancy, that is, until they are faced with caring for a home. The young bride resents the hard work she finds waiting for her as a housewife, when her unpreparedness for this work has made her so responsive to glittering promises. In the dizzy race to make life "easy—easier—easiest" is a time coming when your living will be done altogether for you?

Despite the discrepancy between promise and fact, the housewife today does benefit immensely from machines. Her kitchen bears little resemblance to the kitchen of a century ago. If the young housewife today could look into the past and watch her grandmother go about her household tasks, she might realize that little is expected in comparison. After seeing her grandmother work over the old coal stove, she would think her assignment small in preparing vegetables for the pressure cooker. Running a vacuum cleaner would be tame compared with the operation accomplished by a straw broom and wet newspaper.

But there were pleasures in the old and now forgotten ways of running a house. The kitchen was a warm and fragrant place. It had to be, as the center of the home and the base for all homemaking. On one wall the coal stove burned almost continuously, and there was usually something simmering there night and day. Vegetables were brought in fresh from the garden, potatoes with the earth clinging to their skins and lettuce with dew between its leaves. The kitchen was a comfortable place to work, and a comfortable place for the family to gather. On certain days the air was enriched by the smell of freshly baked bread.

It is time to realize that we must pay for what we gain. Nothing is without its price. What price, then has the machine age exacted upon the mother? It has, in some degree, robbed her of an opportunity for creative work. Is creating not the purpose of living, and does creation not carry with itself its satisfactions and rewards? When women received their freedom, when they gained leisure to follow intellectual interests, they sacrificed the opportunity creatively to express their love for their families.

I have placed a portion of the responsibility on advertising. But this is just the end of a chain of causes. The beginning must be with the woman herself. A woman who enjoyed her work could not so easily be swayed from that enjoyment by pictures and slogans in a magazine.

There is no reason why housework cannot be aided by machines, and yet allow a great deal of room for creative work. There should be even greater pleasure in cooking a meal on a new gas range than on the coal stove. And the steam iron can do a better job on ruffles and pleats than the clumsy metal contrivance of the past.

The hard labor of our grandmothers can by no stretch of the imagination have been more enjoyable than the house-wife's work today. We need not doubt how happy (however, also frightened) a farm wife of the last century would have been, had she found herself suddenly transported to a twentieth-century kitchen. The woman who receives the bene-fits of such projects as that of the Tennessee Valley Authority must consider herself in a man-made paradise.

But these women knew the art of working with their hands. Labor-saving devices could only enhance their *direct experi-ence* of providing for their families. They scrubbed floors on their hands and knees, and they knew the texture of kneaded bread, they prepared food, not by precisely measured recipe but critical and appreciative tasting. Through the work they performed their senses were keen. By their own physical effort they met the challenge of caring for their loved ones. And no labor-saving devices could make them forget the satisfactions of that direct experience. Many "recipes" dif-fused through an eager public today are but poor ersatz ver-sions of the things lost.

But how are women today to know this satisfaction? The machine will not help them learn. A woman must know the pleasure of her work before she can increase that pleasure by the aid of appliances. The pre-packaged dinner will never bring the praise from her family that was evoked in an earlier time by the homemade original, beef stew and apple pie, even though the ad assures her that her "husband tastes the home-made flavor." But she does not know her loss. And so, all that remains for her, despite the aid technology has extended, is the tedious side of housework.

Gradually, women are realizing that their work in the home offers opportunity for creative expression. Some women are beginning to bake their own bread. Advertisers, recognizing this trend, have adapted some of their offers to it. There are now rolls that require the last baking touch at home, cakes so advanced in their preparation that by just putting them in

255

the oven the illusion of skillful home baking will be attained. It remains that the most significant sign of woman's recognition of their own and their families' needs is that they have been turning away from jobs and careers and, in increasing numbers, returning to their homes.

Though it has eased their work, the machine age has robbed men, as well, of opportunity to work with their hands. From their need to have the *direct experience* of handling materials have arisen basement workshops, do-it-yourself kits, and innumerable hobbies. Men who spend their days working in offices with abstract figures and ideas have reacted by filling their leisure hours with these undertakings. But it is not enough that they be used for diversion. Direct experience with its trail of satisfactions should be brought back into the working day as well. Or else the same man who is an addict of do-it-yourself kits may find himself powerless before a simple mechanical breakdown in his house, able only to call the handy man.

The girl who is unacquainted with housework has little chance of enjoying that work when she marries. However light it be compared with the past, it will hold no satisfactions for her. In this area, as in others, she has lost *the pleasure of direct experience*.

In no area has woman lost so much as in the care of her baby. Modern devices and opinions have combined to keep the mother unaware of the joy that a close contact with her baby would bring. We see a reaction to this in the work of Ribble.[2] Breast feeding is a striking example. The satisfactions it affords to mother and child have been almost forgotten in this age of bottles and formulas. In recent years it has been held as obsolete, a little ridiculous, and the young mother who dared go counter to the prevailing custom felt the need to apologize. It was not many years ago that the doctors went so far as to warn women against it. By some strange logic they argued that it was easier to wean a baby from a bottle than from the breast. But behind the doctor's warnings, behind the rationalizations, there again lie the feelings of the woman herself. She was unwilling to sacrifice her time to her baby. An unconscious expression of this unwillingness was translated for many mothers in inadequate milk secretion.

One conviction gradually yields to another. Women today are again beginning to nurse their babies, some following the advice of their doctors, some resistive to medical injunction. But breast feeding will not have its full value until mothers can enjoy it, enjoy the physical closeness of their baby, and allow their baby the serenity and security of contact with his mother's body.

A mother who is unable to nurse her baby might reach the same closeness in many other ways. But these too have been lost in a time when sterilized bottles and scientifically prepared formulas have become more important than time spent with the baby. A mail order house promised the mother the last step to freedom from her child—a goose-neck bottle holder that could be attached to the crib. It must be added that this awe-inspiring armature did not meet with the anticipated commercial success. In more recent years it has been replaced by playful animals which hold the bottle with a grin, and for all their playfulness remain impersonal and unmotherly. No further comment is necessary to point out the magnitude of this custom reflected here and its import.

Babies, like other people, have their likes and dislikes. Many mothers fail to recognize their individualities and to cater to their tastes. In a time gone by the mother would have her baby in the kitchen while she was cooking. She might feed him tidbits that appealed especially to him. Free from worry over formula and prepared and measured baby foods, she guided her baby's diet according to his taste and his eventual selection by taste preference. We know now that small children do not go far wrong even in their ignorance of calories and vitamins. The child grew, knowing the enjoyment of food.

Today the baby is brought up on a balanced diet, scientifically approved as better than the easy-going fare of his predecessor. He may be assured of the correct dosage of vitamins. He will start eating solid foods at the right moment. But his mother will probably not have time to pay attention to what he wants, in her concern over what he needs. This baby will lose the pleasure and security of enjoying tempting food as he sits in the comfort of his mother's lap.

Discipline can be a great problem for the mother who is

not close to her child. She will have to rely on rules, and rules change with disconcerting frequency. At one moment the anxious mother will be warned to use firm discipline. At the next she will be told to allow her child complete freedom. Suppression will then be the great evil. Today the policy is one of compromise, defined by the word "permissive." But this is not an easy policy to follow. It does not demand, as some interpreters would have it, complete indulgence. It asks rather for a balance of freedom for experiment with support from authority figures. To control his desires by consideration for others as well as by the limits of reality the child needs support and guidance from his parents. It will give him the security he needs and can find in the love of parents, who know and can give limits in situations where license can arouse guilt feelings.

Because permissiveness is not easy, it is generally allowed to become over-indulgence by parents. In order to apply discipline wisely it is necessary to know a child, to understand him and his needs. It is necessary to see things from his point of view. For we seldom stop to realize that the world through the eyes of a child is a large and bewildering place. Not that the child is unable to let his feelings be known. Revealing comments from him are voiced, though not heard. Too often, if heard, they become sources of amusement, not information.

Numerous are the tracts, pamphlets, and books written on the subject of permissive discipline. But can it be taught as a science? If there is between mother and child a bond of love and understanding, then the mother will be led by her feelings to give her child the amount of guidance and the kind of guidance that he needs. But if there is no bond, if the mother has not shared her child's joys and disappointments from his early years, she can hardly hope to reach him later. And the choice is not entirely up to her. For her relation with her child has been molded by her own relation to her mother. If she has received warm understanding as a child, that understanding will not fail her as a mother. Benjie's mother in *Children of Divorce*[3] was proof of this patterning after a mother-image.

There is no break in the link of mother-child relationships.

The fate of the family rests upon the mother. Her capacity to give love, or the lack of it, will give strength or weakness to her children. And they will pass on what they have received from her to their own children.

A child's relation with society is determined to the largest extent by his mother. For his mother first introduces him to society, she forms his first contact with the world, and at first, his only contact. Birth does not sever him from complete dependence on her. He remains physically dependent, and, more important, emotionally dependent. If he receives simple and warm love from his mother, his path toward emotional maturity will be smoothed. But if her love is inadequate, or if it is complicated by her own emotional conflicts, then this will be difficult indeed. Thus, in her relation to the world and her relation to her child the mother will play a uniquely important part in his development and behavior.

Perhaps this sounds very final. There is room for later correction. Even though personality development takes shape during the child's very early years, it can always be reshaped to some degree, but with some limitations already set. Emotional conflicts can be worked through. Maternal love may not be the magic formula against all emotional ills, but surely it is more important than any other influence. For in the early years the nucleus of neurosis and mental illness may be formed in a child; and the greatest protection a child can have during these years is love.

It is necessary to stress this again and again, because we are notably lacking today in mothers who are able to express their love. To what extent this paucity can be related to the age in which we live—this cannot be measured in decibels or drams, but its effects are legible in many present-day problems of children's emotional adjustments. Our mechanized age has divorced us from many direct experiences, and among them one of the most important: the experience of a close relation between mother and child.

How is the boy today helped toward adulthood? Our ideal of manhood is presented to him at every turn. This is the "he-man" ideal. The "he-man" lives by an individualistic code (with a shadow of conformism backstage), a code protecting the rights of the weak and asserting his strength against his equals. Towards women he shows gentleness, but his weapon against men is brute strength.

The mother of a boy cannot escape the pressure of this much wonted ideal. It is impressed upon her through popular literature and radio and television with their made-to-order heroes. If she is immature, she may not be able to prevent it from assuming significance out of all proportion. If so, her child's development will reflect her vulnerability.

Compulsive training, rigid eating patterns, and other pressures on her part lead her to making her boy a man without delay. If he is not inclined to kick back an aggressive playmate, she will anxiously accuse him of being a sissy. Pushing him away before he is ready, she will try to shame him into standing up for his own rights. Not only will she encourage him to be aggressive, but she will try to speed up his growth in other ways. And always this conflict between the easy way of *laissez faire* and the press of rushing him to conform to the rigid standards set by our culture.

Such a mother gets results. But does she realize exactly what these results are? Her boy, unable to stand ridicule and shame, develops early the protective outward shell of a man. Fearing himself a sissy, he hides his fears under a cover of bravado. Within lurks the frightened little boy. But this remains well concealed. When he carried it to an extreme, he develops into the bully, and then into the difficult boy who feels the need to assert himself in "manly" ways. The forbidden cigarette, the hot rod and whiskey put in a precocious appearance. His reckless and antisocial attitudes are but part of his ill-fitting garments of manhood. Underneath is the child who has lost the opportunity for normal growth.

Gorer[4] has reminded us that men in America are often referred to as "little boys," or as "great big babies." Behind these expressions, sometimes of fondness, sometimes ridicule, lies the realization of the serious fact that the immature boy remains within many a man. In emergencies this may become apparent in disastrous fashion. For it was reflected in the numerous breakdowns which took place under the stress of war, even after careful screening at induction.

Such men fail not only under stress. They are often sexual failures as well. This is but another facet of their incomplete and disturbed emotional development, as a result of a dependency on the mother which they have not outgrown. Many men today still feel the need for a protection and love which they did not receive as children. Unable to give the mature love demanded by marriage, they unconsciously expect from their wives what they did not have from their mothers. Their marriages are doomed to failure—a reminder that one of three marriages ends in divorce.

The mother is not the only important influence on the growing boy. The father may, to an extent, make up for poor maternal relationship. But this is unlikely. What can the father himself contribute if, as is possible, he has had the same maternal influence in his own early years? How many fathers today are emotionally strong enough to offer their sons a satisfactory image for identification? From one generation to the next the mother demands of her son a premature masculinity which stunts his emotional growth, and from one generation to the next we can count on strong, hefty, but immature men.

And what of the girl in this family group? How is she affected by the lack of warm maternal love? The consequences are far-reaching, since her own deprivation will be reflected in the bringing up of her children, either as deficiency or overcompensation, one not more healthful than the other. Her destiny and that of the next generation are stamped.

The "ideal woman" in America is difficult of formulation. Suppose we imagine her to be the mother and homemaker type. And suppose her daughter is patterned after this ideal. When she reaches her teens, she will find herself a misfit in her social group. While her gayer, more glamourous friends enjoy great social success, she will remain the wallflower. Boys are seldom interested in girls with the flavoring of a homemaker and mother. We know what a fetish is made of glamour, a Hollywood- and T.V.-shaped fantasy, yet so real and absorbing to teenagers. On the other hand, emotionally tied as they are to their mothers, boys are unconsciously attracted to a motherly type of person, in apparent contradiction with their readiness to get caught in the trappings of the glamour girl.

Not many girls will be found struggling under the delusion

that being a homemaker will assure them of finding desirable husbands, and they will soon have to concede to glamour. If not many girls are found to be avid for rich, full home-making, it is because there are fewer and fewer mothers to point the way. Generalizations are always dangerous, but an all-inclusive survey is not in line here. However, two groups of mothers deserving comment stand out. There is the over-anxious mother, uncertain of herself, torn between the varying do's and don't's of this school of discipline and that. There is the other, the immature woman who cannot face the responsi-bility of being a parent, turning rather to the carefree pleasure-seeking that is typical of the adolescent. Neither of these mothers can set a well-focused image for their daughters to follow.

As she grows up the girl will find herself in additional con-fusion while trying to establish her place in the family and so-ciety. Her father's position can hardly escape her. Undoubtedly she will recognize the little boy that resides in the so-called head of the family. She will see his dependence on her mother, and yet it will be asked of her to accept woman's nominal in-feriority. Her brother and her father are built up as powerful structures, despite the fact that she senses their weakness as opposed to her mother's strength.

Some schools of psychiatry have offered as fundamental her penis-envy conflict. Whether considered instinctual or cultural, the dynamics are at work. She can scarcely know to what sex she belongs. A frequent escape nowadays is an early marriage, to the world and to herself evidence of her womanliness. This is, of course, a futile escape. Frigidity, among other failures, will reveal her emotional conflicts.

As an alternate she may turn to sexual experimentation and activities. There are alarming reports of increase in this area, an increase which has been blamed on the widespread use and approval of birth control, and the ease with which contraceptives can be purchased. But the mere removal of the fear of pregnancy is not at the root of the matter. Emotional insecurity and confusion lead to precocious sex stimulation and promiscuity among young people. A healthy restraint is based on sound emotional development. How many mothers are mature enough and loving enough to provide their daughters with that valuable fund? Thus, not a few girls are deprived of the emotional background that leads to happy adult life.

The girl's problem today is highlighted by certain extreme cases, including juvenile delinquency and severe mental disorders. To illustrate, a group of delinquent girls who were at the New York State Training School for Girls were studied in 1947.[5] Larger and more intensive studies by the Gluecks[6, 7] have brought out many interesting facts, a small aspect of which is being considered here. The comparison of delinquent girls with girls suffering from mild emotional conflicts, while it needs to be qualified, is enlightening.

Although the newspapers remind us daily of the alarming increase in juvenile delinquency (and from whatever vantage point you look there is an increase) the proportion of our population so recognized by law is not as sensational as headlines flash it. Request for examination of these girls was made because of the special problems they presented at the New York State Training School and because they suffered from severe emotional problems. Their story is thus heavily weighted. Allowing for the artifact, theirs remains a grim example of the ends to which a troubled mother-daughter relationship can lead.

Their histories were varied, but one theme remains constant. Their relation to their mothers was very disturbed and essentially one of resentment. The mothers themselves were inadequate. A glance through the files shows one case after another of desertion, alcoholism, psychotic disturbances, drug addiction. Many of these mothers were unmarried. Some had abandoned their daughters, and those who remained with them rejected them emotionally.

These girls, almost without exception, responded violently to their mothers' indifference. Their resentment varied from sullen coldness to outright hatred. In contrast to their lack of love for their mothers they, one and all, showed a tendency to ally themselves with their fathers, a desire to identify with them, even when their feelings were ambivalent.

What sort of men were they to inspire this feeling in their daughters? Only two out of the whole group could be considered reasonably healthy fathers from the emotional point

263

of view. The remainder were alcoholics, deserters, law-breakers of various types, unstable personalities, or unknown altogether.

Inadequacies were in both parents. But the girls were prone to put all blame and responsibility on their mothers. Without objective justification they continued to trust in their fathers. They explained away their fathers' failures. One girl, who spoke bitterly of her mother, said of her father, "He got the same rotten break I did." Another girl, typical of many, would not believe that her father had deserted her. She continued to send him letters, although she never received an answer. She could not face the fact that her father would never again be part of her home.

In identifying with their fathers these girls assumed masculine attitudes. They walked with a swagger and assumed masculine posture and stance. Homosexuality was rampant in the institution.

What has this to do with girls from a "normal" background? Their emotional confusion can hardly lead to these extremes. Nevertheless, their stories are parallel. They show a strong attachment to their fathers and reject their mothers, because of the latter's failure to give love.

This type of woman is often very successful in business. From her rank are drawn many famous career women. Trouble is brought home when she marries and has a family. Then her womanliness fails her. Her manliness may not be discernible in her appearance. Many a gentle voice and frilly attire are only thin veils over masculine assertiveness.

Generally, she will not be troubled in competing with her husband, for she will instinctively choose him from among those men who lack aggressive masculine qualities. She will have the sensitivity and find the little boy under the tough exterior of the man she marries. The pattern then is almost invariable. Marrying an emotionally weak man, she will proceed to overwhelm and weaken the children—an unconscious pattern, not a willful and deliberate design.

Her daughters will have little chance for normal growth. Their mother's emotional story before them, they may become defeminized. Or, sensing her rejection, they will turn to their fathers. There too will they find little emotional support. They can hardly escape one form of neuroticism or another.

Strecker was the first to describe these mothers clinically,[8] incorporating this concept into the psychiatric literature and thought. It has since become widely recognized. Philip Wylie, using the novelist's privilege of imaginative overstatement, has made this woman famous in a portrait which he labels "The American Mom."[9]

The story of the "American Mom" is not a happy one, neither for her children nor for herself, not to mention her husband. A changing and confusing society has weighed heavily on the individual mother and wife. The neuroticism passes down from children to grandchildren. Are her sons developing fully as men? Her daughters certain of their womanliness? To her and to the husband of her choice will be born children who are torn between the roles of boy and girl, and later—man and woman. This is an almost inescapable outcome.

THE FRAGMENTS AND THE WHOLE

America today is dedicated to the young. As nowhere else in the world, children enjoy a carefree existence and the pursuit of pleasure. To them fall none of the responsibilities which burden their contemporaries elsewhere. Happiness for them is our goal, for, we reason, all too soon must they relinquish it to take up the cares and drudgeries of adult life.

Youth is our dream and our idea. And thus, adulthood can be little but disillusionment, awakening to harsh reality. Little wonder it is that ours is a century of so many neurotic adults, adults living in confusion and anxiety, looking back upon the dream of their youth and fearing the future. Uncertain of themselves, they are anxious to provide their children with the happiness that seems to have eluded them.

We see to it that our children have the best physical care available. Not only are they provided with fresh vegetables, meat, milk, and bread in quantity. But the bread is enriched with niacin and iron, the milk with vitamin D. Our teachers see to it that respective families are, via pupils, duly informed of the minimum diet requirement. Pills are absorbed in bewildering variety, mothers carefully adding these to their children's already rich diet. Mail order catalogues with pages of listed vitamin products keep up with the latest discoveries applicable to geriatrics, pediatrics, and plain everyday, everybody's needs.

Such abundance would overwhelm most of our European neighbors. So too would the houses that shelter the majority of American families. Children here for the great part live in suburban dream worlds, worlds of compact houses activated by the latest that gadgetry can provide. Electricity and hot water are to be had at the press of a button or the turn of a tap. Even as our children enjoy the convenience of modern living, children of the same age in Europe and elsewhere have existed in a war-damaged world, a world where the majority of families survived at the minimum subsistence level.

The child of these shores has not always enjoyed the privileges now bestowed upon him. His lot, even then in Colonial times, was not as hard as that of the children just mentioned. Nevertheless, centuries of neglect and submission must have stirred up guilt in parents. The rebellion of children, exploding in the American Child Revolution, left parents powerless because of these very guilt feelings. Victims turned judges.

Do we feel so guilty about our own children that we feel compelled to give everything money can provide? Today it is the twenty-five-cent allowance so that our son has as much as the boy next door. Tomorrow it will be a bicycle because his friend has one. The demands do not lessen, they increase. Soon he will have to have the use of the family car, or a car of his own. It was not long ago that a noted educator was quoted at length in an advertisement for television, saying that children without television sets must be considered "underprivileged." It attests to the sanity of parents that this debt to children was heartily protested. But the slack has been taken up. If a child today hears of another unfortunate enough not to have a set, his heart swells in pity and bewilderment.

Parents hesitate to offer criticism of their child's efforts, relying on the belief that youngsters benefit from encouragement and laudatory affluence. If Mary's first piece of clay sculpture suffers from a wobbly formlessness, her parents would be the last to suggest improvement. As far as Mary knows, she has nothing further to learn of the art of sculpting. And how unfair to Mary!

All children need to feel secure. Many parents find that the easiest way to give their children this security is by sheltering them from unpleasant realities of family life. Problems are concealed, particularly those concerning money. Many an American father works himself ragged to provide his children with the best toys, summer camp, and with all those things his friends have. Better to buy a second car or a television set on the installment plan than to disturb the child with the thought that his father is not as well off as his neighbor.

Many parents feel that responsibilities will come to their children soon enough, that their children must enjoy unrestrained freedom and pleasure in abundance. Neither work nor family problems should be a part of a child's life. His proper function being to enjoy himself, it is up to the parents to see that he does. This goes against the child's instinct. He wants to be part of everything, even as he cannot encompass his own physical limitations. Witness the nursery school child who races busily with his pointed announcement to the world, "I've got some work to do."

At what point will the child make a transition from childhood to maturity? What stroke of magic will turn him from complete self-centeredness to a sense of responsibility toward others? When will his ego be considered strong enough to accept the reality of effort to an end, with its satisfaction and accomplishment? It is during the teens that most parents expect a change, or realize the need for it. It is then they note with consternation that their son, although he stands a head taller than his father, still behaves like a child when he cannot have his own way. They may try last-minute measures of discipline and angrily lay down rules. Their daughter now uses lipstick and wears high heeled shoes, and yet she throws her clothes around her room as she did when she was a child. When told to come in at a certain time in the evening, she answers with a temper tantrum or deception. No amount of pleading, of shouting, can turn this girl into a responsible, emotionally mature person. Now in his teens the adolescent's natural desire to be rid of parental restraints resonates with the long-known indulgence. The child is unleashed into an unmanageable young adult.

When self-discipline has not been learned in slow, gradual steps from childhood on, it cannot be expected to flourish suddenly during the teen-age years. For this is the period when the child feels the greatest need to reject all authority and face the world on his own. And so it is that many adolescents create standards entirely their own, in a world where sloppy clothes constitute a uniform, where a special language is spoken that excludes all outsiders. Their pleasures may range from jitterbug and mambo, harmless in themselves, to hard drinking, fast driving, marijuana, and various degrees of sex experimentation. When attempting to write of these hectic waves it is futile to try and catch up with the latest fad. The mass reaction to these fast-moving waves is an index of the vulnerability of the immature adolescent. A sixteen-year-old girl must find emotional satisfaction from copying the latest hairdo of a starlet and live by proxy every instant of her daily and intimate life. The posthumous obsession with James Dean illustrates the point. An eighteen-year-old boy, poorly tied up to his own everyday reality, plagues his parents for a car, an escape from his emotional vacuum and an instrument of power which will make him the "big shot" to his pals (not his friends, he has none). The "hot rod" is on its way to mowing down its quota of victims.

These, it will be admitted, are the extremes of teen-age behavior. But even though most of their pleasures are harmless, the majority of these youngsters are faced with a grave problem. This year they are still children. But tomorrow will follow, and tomorrow they will be adults.

While the boy's desire to get away from home may be a carefree one at first, it will soon be a required part of getting a job and marrying. The girl who has enjoyed the "grown-up" pleasure of nylons and lipstick will soon be called upon to take on the responsibility of being a wife and mother. Will the boy, suddenly with a wife and job, be able to find happiness in the unexpected demands made upon him, demands for which he has not been prepared? Will the girl see anything but hard labor in her daily tasks as housewife and mother? The figures on divorce—well known in its legal form, unfathomable in its emotional form—give us part of the answer.

The experience of growing up in a family where worries and pleasures are shared, where family responsibilities are shouldered by everyone, builds in a child a deep sense of belonging and makes for the kind of *communication* within the family which is so lacking today. Felt early, this sense of belonging will, through the vicissitudes of later years, afford a sturdiness which is irreplaceable.

Our children, to a great extent, are sheltered from family life. They grow up exposed to the myth of "golden youth." This myth lies behind our advertising, our popular literature, our entertainment. Women are encouraged to retain their youth at all cost. They are lauded for growing younger every day. Mothers, grandmothers, they would everlastingly remain "the girls." Beauty experts promise youth; musical comedies glorify it. The middle-aged man looks back with nostalgia on his school days, eagerly awaiting college reunions when he can recapture his boyhood freedom by frolicking and playing the clown.

The teen-ager cannot be expected to look forward to the pleasures of adult life, when his parents take so little satisfaction in them, or, at least, fail, if they have any, to share their satisfaction with him. He has probably heard from his parents, from his relatives, even from his graduation speaker in high school, that the days of his youth are the happiest of his life, and that anxious and weary times lie ahead. Today the teen-ager already knows the pleasures of adulthood in some of their more easily accessible paths, drinking, smoking, and sex. All that seems to remain is hard work and the care of a family and job. Is the expectancy worth the trepidation?

O. Spurgeon English, clinical professor of psychiatry at Temple University Medical School, defined this teen-age attitude in an address to the American Academy of General Practice, in 1952. He called it the "emotional undernourishment of teen-agers." The situation he describes is a common one.

> A visit to the home will all too often show the teen-age daughter watching television or talking to a friend while the mother is overworked and the house is in disorder. This teen-age daughter has the early symptoms of a social illness known as marital unhappiness which often ends in the unpleasant operation of divorce.

Where does this girl learn her dislike for homemaking and its necessary adjunct, housework? Probably from her mother, who, by her own example, has made housework seem unrewarding drudgery.

Before this lack of family cohesion children are quick to force themselves into a tyrannical position. Not only do they seldom offer help to their parents, even less seek their counsel and guidance, but they often feel it necessary to correct their parents and instruct them. In the same meeting at which Dr. English spoke on the teen-age girl, Dr. Richard A. Kern of Temple University remarked that teen-agers today felt obliged to "raise their parents."

Where does this teen-age authority and domination originate? It has not always been so. Let us not forget the centuries of oblivion and abject neglect and the violent rebellion of the American Child Revolution, followed by the tightening up of the Victorians. It is extremely unlikely that a fourteen-year-old in our grandfather's time would have corrected his father, or expressed disapproval about his old-fashioned ways. If such thoughts entered his mind, they would have remained unspoken. But it is likely that children of the last century did not entertain these thoughts. Early repression dealt with them effectively. Their parents represented an unquestioned, reliable authority. Today parents, in their uncertainty, invite their children's disquietude. With little confidence in oneself, is it possible to emanate a feeling of inner strength?

The insecurity of parents in our time is exemplified in the wavering handling of their children and reflected in the various trends in child training of the last decade or so. Not only have parents trusted in the advice of child experts gathered from magazine, radio, and television, but the new expert's advice conflicts with that of the last, and the followers, dutifully marching into step, lose their direction. Yesterday's mother anxiously left her baby in his crib to cry. Today's mother rushes to cuddle him at the slightest whimper. Yesterday's mother fretted and fussed early over her child's toilet habits, training him as soon as he could sit, or before. Today's mother may neglect such training until it has become an all too obvious necessity, perhaps until kindergarten. Not long ago children were spanked at the least provocation. Today such spanking will be considered damaging. At one moment comic books are snatched fearfully from children, in dread that they will be led straight to juvenile delinquency. At the next moment these same comic books are eulogized as a normal outlet for the child's aggressive feelings. There is no end to the train of contradictory do's and don't's in child care. The mother who rushes from one to another will be at a loss to gain confidence and respect from her child, for she does not have that confidence in herself. He need not be acquainted with the sources to sense her lack of stability.

Expert advice is not given without reservations and special qualifications. The experts know that child psychology is a groping science with only part of the answers available. But, in their uncertainty, parents are prone to rush for new solutions without reserve of critical appraisal, and without measuring them in terms of their own child's particular needs. To them the word is Gospel. But though it becomes a golden rule for these parents, it is, nevertheless, a momentary one.

The multiplicity of advice in the absence of a grasp of general principles, moreover, can be dangerous: one thousand situations can be conjured up and a solution be given for each, but the one thousand and first situation emerges which has not been anticipated. No ready formula is within reach, and the parent is lost. Advice must remain general and flexible to be functional and apply to each individual.

Facts and figures change very little. But, depending on the commentator followed, these facts and figures tell very different stories at different times. One moment they are used to support the conclusion that our teen-age world is one of alcoholics, drug addicts, gang leaders, and murderers. At the next moment the same figures are used to convince us that the child today is happy, productive, and well on the way to becoming the well-adjusted citizen of tomorrow, with only a few exceptions to check the rule.

Many parents would be startled and resentful to be told that they do not know their children. Having lavished everything upon them, sparing nothing to provide them with education and all the advantages of modern recreation and pleasure, they do not realize that they have, nevertheless, failed really to know them.

Not that they have not tried. To just such an audience go copy after copy of books on child training, magazines, and newspaper articles. But the more doggedly they pursue these sources of information, the more do they lose sight of the child they seek to understand. A revealing way of referring to her child has recently crept into the everyday vocabulary of the modern mother. "My two-year-old," or "my five-year-old," are words which, for what they represent, make one cringe. A category, a prototype, a schema of behavior and achievements useful to the psychologists and pediatricians who have tabulated means and averages. Why is it used—so literally—by the mother to substitute for "my baby," or "my daughter," or "my little boy"?

Parents are overwhelmed and confused by facts and figures which they are unable adequately to use in their attempts to understand their child and establish a two-way communication. This undermines their confidence as parents. Psychiatric experience with children drives this point home forcefully. Numerous illustrations could be given. Here is one.

The parents of a twelve-year-old boy bring him to the attention of a psychiatrist. Very briefly, his history is one of long standing illnesses which are neurotically determined, but have been interpreted on an entirely physical basis. The boy when first seen describes his symptoms with a terminology which immediately reveals a delusional character. He speaks of "ants and bugs crawling inside my chest." Since no physical illness could produce such a body sensation, there can be no misinterpretation of the symptom. However, when informed of the severity of the illness (one very small facet of which is given here for illustration) the parents insisted that the boy had freely "always talked about everything, and why shouldn't he tell us that also?" A child's early painful experiences, overlooked by the parents in their own account of the child's history, expressions of feelings altogether unsuspected by them, emerge during a first interview. This challenge of the first interview with a child is one invariably encountered. Parents are shocked and bewildered suddenly to realize that their child can "reveal" on initial contact some inner feelings that they had not at any point been aware of.

This is the child psychiatrist's experience. However, let any doubt be dispelled that only parents of emotionally disturbed children are thus alienated.

Why should a child be such a mystery to his parents? In part, as we have seen, it is that adults block their memories of early years, but there is again the lack of communication—here and now. There is no easy path toward the understanding of another. Human relations demand something more than just time and effort. Feelings will carry one much farther than the intellect.

Parents cannot expect to have the knowledge and training of the psychologist or psychiatrist. Nor should they wish for them. They need not interpret motives or analyze situations. But, if they are close to their child, they have the answer to many of their questions. Such closeness—a closeness which begins at birth, let us recall—is often lost amid the child study that occupies parents today.

Problems, mostly minor ones, invariably come up in dealing with children, and these problems take shape in relation to the individual child, though they be recognized in a class or type. Mary may seem a normally aggressive little girl, ready to join in with any game her friends devise, eager always for some new adventure, a new school, a new camp, a new home. But her brother, Peter, may be quite a different person. He may have difficulty making friends, preferring whenever possible to retire to a world of his own in books and hobbies. The suggestion of summer camp may send him into tears. If Peter's parents are close to him, if they understand him as a person, they will learn that he needs more loving than Mary, whose personal attractiveness he may resent, that he needs special encouragement and support, that he needs to be drawn out. His parents need no books to grasp this, if they know their son. If they don't, attempts to analyze his behavior, to classify it under a terminology which has little or no meaning to them, even though it may have been popularized over the airwaves, all such attempts will be futile and, indeed, can only further separate them from their child. It isn't knowledge itself that is under criticism, but knowledge without feeling.

A child psychiatrist's experience highlights this point. In first contact with parents of an emotionally disturbed child great pain is taken initially to indicate that the psychiatrist is not interested in any opinion, professional or otherwise, on

274

the child brought for observation. Would the parents tell, not what Dr. — or Miss — (teacher) thinks is the trouble with the youngster, but only what it is that they, the parents, are troubled about and for which they are now seeking help. Despite this pointed preparation, answers are frequently of the order, "She has an inferiority complex. . . . I think he has a split personality. . . . His behavior is too aggressive for his age . . . etc."

Minor problems, if overlooked early, tend to grow in intensity and complexity. At this stage can the attentive parents' help be most effective. If they are close to their son, they cannot miss the small signs of emotional dissonance. The young boy will not have trouble in later years, if his parents help him past his difficulties now. But if they are out of touch with him, his problem becomes so complex and so foreign to them that only a skilled person will be able to recognize it and help resolve it. And even this is not guaranteed. Often a mother who has missed this early communication tends to switch her attention to the child's physical needs.

It may be necessary at this time to clarify two concepts which are frequently confused, independence and remoteness. They are unwarrantedly taken for equivalents. In striving to give independence to their children too early, parents may be fostering a detachment which their child feels as a sort of rejection. Emotional separation, which is part of the maturation process, is not best achieved through parental remoteness. Indeed, such a remoteness tends to increase desire for dependence (clinging), or, to the contrary, bring about an affective withdrawal on the part of the child—a withdrawal which is not conducive to healthy emotional development.

Here is a striking example of the kind of remoteness under discussion. A father, troubled about his son, brought a complete record of the boy, volumes of it, thrusting them on the desk as his first gesture. This was the result of ten years of careful filing of photographs, dates, comments. This was his son, month by month, year by year. He was capable of looking at the boy with an objective detachment truly alarming. It was little more than the record of a laboratory worker noting the actions and reactions of an anthropoid under observation. Although it was had later, no interview with the boy was needed to tell that he was suffering from a deep emotional disturbance. The child, his feelings, the interrelations within the family or among outside groups, did not live through the mass of notations, accurate, incisively detailed. This is an extreme case, not unique.

It has become fashionable to be glibly conversant about the new topic, child psychology. The warm, homey little tales of Johnny's progress, his gauche humor, his spontaneous and unsophisticated wisdom, his astute observations, have no place in the smart abstractions on the child, so familiar to us today.

What a feeling parent will recall of his child's early years may still be accurate, but it has a flavor all its own. He does not say, "my three-year-old walked at one year and ten days, this is about as in the book . . . etc.," rather he recalls the chair and the rug, the place where the father was sitting. He recalls that the mother was leaning toward the child, the wobbly little form making a sudden start, with all the signs of excitement, laughing on the verge of tears, all the light touches which stamped the occasion a memorable date. The date may have slipped temporarily from his mind, but the accuracy of the emotional recall will easily bring back temporal relationships.

The gap which can exist between a child and his parents is not always so wide as in the extreme example of the father and his son as given earlier. In milder form the remoteness and lack of communication between parents and children emotionally disturbed to various degrees is very common.

Here, for instance, is a barely five-year-old little girl, only child of divorced parents. She is brought by her mother to the attention of the psychiatrist, primarily because of the divorce situation. Her parents had been separated from the time she was one and a half. She lives with her mother; her father, whom she recalls from earlier years, now lives several thousand miles away and has visited her at irregular intervals. The mother's formulation of the problem revolved about the puzzling behavior of the little girl, who, on the one hand clung to her, begged her not to go to work or leave the house ever, and on the other hand was negative and showed a great deal of hostility to her mother when sometimes, at the cost of her own adult enjoyments, she stayed home with her child. The mother wanted to know if she was "handling her right. . . . Are there things that should be knocked out of her?" Although she lives in a disorganized and emotionally depriving family unit, one good fortune had this child, that a warm, comfortable, steady Negro maid has been her constant companion since the separation of the parents. There is a very close relationship between the two.

The mother is unable to provide most of the data about the early development of her child. Coming to the focal point of the problem, i.e., the divorce, she reports that the child doesn't ask about her father, having been told that he is thousands of miles away because of his work. One contact with the child brings out a quite different story. True, she has not talked about her father, but she is bewildered about her father living away and comments that "other children see their daddies more often." She would like to see him, "but he's too far away." Why? Because he has to work there, etc. The child, in her next comment, gives away the early sequence of events when the psychiatrist suggests that she could ask Mommy about these things that puzzle her. She says, "I don't know how to ask Mommy. I asked her once. She said her has to work at home."

So there we have a mother who feels that the child does not need to ask, having been satisfied with the "work" answer, and a child who feels that she cannot ask further questions, even though her strange situation, unlike that of others, is bewildering to her. The lack of communication in this picture is self-evident. The fact that the child, considered a fairly normal child, is not emotionally disturbed is obviously due to the fact that she has had a good mother-substitute.

Perhaps we ask too much of parents. Perhaps society's growing complexity has made the task of bringing up children too great for parents alone. Children mature more slowly than in those days when society was simply organized, even though they may give early an impression of sophistication which our age of intense promoting and vulgarization fosters on them. Parents themselves have difficulty in meeting the demands of the world around them. They often feel incapable of facing these changing demands and find themselves helpless in guiding their children through the long process of growth to maturity in such a world.

A few fundamental values, relating, for instance, to the parental role, ego strength, unity and integration of the individual, remain unchallenged by changes, slow or rapid, which are taking place. Within the family these values are nurtured. The loosening up of the structure threatens the fundamental values. One may ask, did the family as a unit gain from material progress or did the losses negate the gains? Much of the sharing which came naturally from the very huddling of the members of the family is lost. Although it is not desirable that it be recaptured in the same form, the emotional loss is, nevertheless, a fact. What is there to take its place?

America is not alone to face this dilemma, and, indeed, it is likely to affect many more countries as modern concepts spread. The English have met the problem in various ways. Recruited for the most part from the ranks of spinsters, the English "nanny," formerly an institution, is by now almost a legend. As a mother-substitute she once played a substantial role in the lives of children of the middle and upper classes. Hers was a familiar and comforting figure in the nursery, presiding over meals, joining in games, reassuring at times of distress. Her charges saw their parents on a formal basis, respected them, indeed were in awe of them, and looked up to them as images of what they themselves must later become. The mother was remote, the father more and more a shadowy figure. It was from "nanny" that they learned the discipline that prepared them to enter public school, the university, and society. We are familiar with accounts of life in the public school of this age. They leave no doubt about the need of self-discipline upon entering public school life, for the discipline applied there must have taxed the strongest of personalities. Orwell in *Such, Such Were the Joys*,[10] and many other English writers evoking their childhood years, have told us of the harsh, in fact sadistic methods used by masters in shaping the personalities of their young pupils. We know that flogging and other forms of physical punishment were not spared.

In the lower classes, while there was no evidence of substitution, the home, nevertheless, experienced in some other form the loss of the mother. A means to provide the child with warmth and affection in the absence of the working mother was the attempt made by the great innovator Susan Isaacs. She established at London University, where she was professor of psychology and education, a department for the training of mother-substitutes. Her program, initiated in 1930, was an indication that the English were early to understand the plight of the child in the modern family.

The needs of the child remain the same through the ages. Both the nanny and the substitute mother minister to these needs. Ideally, they should be fulfilled by mother and father. This is never so clearly brought out as in the divorce situation. It is imperative that both parents provide the affection to strengthen the child emotionally, and the discipline which will enable him to become a happy and useful member of society. The child should be able to turn to them for comfort. No matter what sociological changes may be on their way, this will still hold. Even the Communists, frantically attempting to enslave the family to the state by first destroying its unity, have learned the devastating effects of such a move. The ill-conceived plan was given up and substituted by efforts at restoring the original unity.

The Papa and Mama of England's Victorian age had a confidence in themselves which parents lack today. They were fully aware of their function in society, and no one, including themselves, questioned their authority as parents. This is not a brief for parental authority for its own sake, nor is it a plea for a return to lost values. But the loss must be gauged, and the need for filling in of this loss thoughtfully considered.

Our children must grow up without that stable environment that once was the unified family. They live in a vacillating society with few and uncertain rules of conduct. Their parents are a part of that society and are shaped by it, unsure as they are of the demands made upon them by parenthood.

There are times when a parent is not available and substitutions must be made. The Negro mammy served this purpose, acting the role of the English nanny in a softer, mellower version, more affectionate, if less learned. But the mammy also has vanished into the past. The mother, busy with job, club, P.T.A., or just because she is a full-time working mother, must all too often hand her children over to the part-time maid or the babysitter. Not too frequently are children as fortunate as the five-year-old little girl previously presented who had the benefit of a warm mother-substitute in what would otherwise have been a very destructive family situation.

So convinced has the government in England been of the child's imperative need for his mother that it conceived a plan worth bringing to mention. It was suggested by the Royal Commission on Population[11] that a mother helper be provided to every home with a child under two, and that such facilities should be increased in proportion to the size of the family. Day nurseries and baby-sitting services should be available, not only in emergencies, but as regular aids to the mother. Vacations were planned, also rest homes for working mothers and summer camps for their children. All this was to be subsidized by the government and only those families who had the funds were required to pay.

That the government wished to provide for the health of its people is not what we want to stress, nor that the family services were initiated. What we should note, however, is that a fact was recognized: the family is the most important unit in society, and this unit has to be preserved. There can be no substitute for the family. However small it may be, it is still the best foundation for human relations. It must remain the most stable and strengthening milieu a child is to have.

The individual stands alone today, faced with a confusing number of choices and decisions. Mechanical aids have, ironically, made his life not simpler but more complex. With society's growing intricacy, man has lost his ability to see himself as a whole, to govern himself by familiar standards, however arbitrary these might be.

Machines were conceived to aid man. But they have taken on a life of their own. There is real danger today that they dominate their creators. We feel compelled to make bigger and better tools, and more of them. If there is no need for them, need is created through advertising and other channels for mass influence. This mechanical profusion has played a large part in breaking up man's life into fragments.

We have already seen that parents no longer treat their children as whole individuals. They concern themselves, rather, with isolated parts of the child's existence. As their outlook towards their children is fragmentary, so is their concept of themselves. Their parenthood is one compartment of their living, their life as husband and wife another. Still a third is their place as members of the community. These compartments do not merge. And thus, their family life, for all its separate enlightenments, shows itself to be in the throes of disintegration.

There is no end to the separate enlightenments today. On the serial plan or in twelve easy chapters one is expected to learn How to Make Friends; How to Be Successful, not necessarily as a whole man, but as husband, as a wife, as a club worker, as a party entertainer; How to Achieve a Successful Marriage; How to Be a Successful Parent, a successful adolescent, a successful cub scout, or a successful toddler, etc. If your goal is not as definite as success in any department of living, then you might turn to the more general topics, All About Eating, All About Your Job, All About Dating, etc. In passing, a search for enlightenment on All About Dying has proved fruitless. You are given credit for native, though limited, endowments when offered opportunities on How to Increase Your Willpower, How to Increase Your Charm, Your Word Power, etc. The profusion of topics and the assurance with which they are handled are indicative enough of the conviction that a design for living can be learned by multiple reference and pin-pointed indexing.

Marriage has not escaped departmentalization. Marriage, which represents the fulfillment of the desire for the richest and most complete human relationship, is not always entered in this spirit. There are today, as always, various reasons for getting married. And any one of them may plunge young people all too quickly into what is meant to be a life-time partnership that should be built on a foundation of love. The reason may be a desire for independence, a means of escape from parents and an opportunity for self-assertion. Or perhaps, unknowingly, marriage may be entered as the only way to appease guilt feelings which would arise from premature sexual relations. Or it may be the seeking of economic security. Marriage may be a direction to follow when nothing else

281

beckons, the socially accepted path for the young person who is through with school.

While the process of dichotomy may be seen in human relations, it is perhaps even clearer in its effects on the professions. A general practitioner, even in rural districts, is no longer a familiar figure in family living. He tends to be a specialist in some branch of medicine. The physicist may know little of the other sciences, and he may know only one small and specialized branch of physics, nuclear physics, electro-magnetics, and so on. Even the younger person, still in college, not yet steered toward a profession, is not given a wide and well-integrated education, aimed at giving some understanding of the whole of man. He may almost immediately take up the study of literature, divorced from history, science, philosophy. And he may soon further specialize in the literature of a single country and a limited period.

Subject specialization as a parody of "research" starts early. In earnest, a bright nine-year-old boy announces that he has some research to do. One is intrigued to hear this word as part of a fourth grader's vocabulary. What is this research about? "Socrates" is the answer, shot out with phonetic uncertainty. It is clear that the boy has no conception of whether this represents a definite point on the earth, or a section of time, or perhaps some strange object which cannot be categorized. Well, how will he do his research? It is with great assurance that he lists his reference sources: the *Encyclopaedia Britannica* and the *Book of Knowledge*. He will write his report on an entity unrelated to the history of philosophy, nor for that matter would he have the faintest glimpse of what a philosopher is. Nevertheless, this boy will go through subsequent years of school learning with the growing satisfaction and the illusion that the picking-out gesture is an act of integration.

Parenthood has also gone the ways of exquisite specialization. It has a literature of its own. With a flip of the finger out of a thorough indexed list, the specific item stands in front of the reader. Read it and you have your solution.

An indexed volume is convenient. But that is not all. There are easier approaches. Daily, parents find themselves directly addressed through newspaper columns or the radio about well-established categories in which, it is assumed, their child fits. "Your three-year-old . . . your eight-year-old . . . your teen-ager." If he doesn't fit, just a little push and he will.

The child in the abstract is much more popular today than the child in the flesh. There is a great deal of interest in the problems of children and childhood, as witnessed by much publicized movements to reform education, to provide under-privileged children with forms of recreation, to deal with juvenile delinquency, drug addiction, etc. Many parents are active in these movements. In dealing with their own chil-dren's demands, their children gradually have slipped out of their hands. The outsider, the school-teacher, the group leader, have taken over part-time.

True, in infancy the child gets total parental attention. Part-time attention, which needs subsequently to be given, actually demands more participation, emotional and intellec-tual, from the parents. This is how a vital communication develops. The bond created between mother and child in the early years will see them both through this kind of communi-cation—a communication which grows daily in substance and complexity. Under the guise of giving freedom to the child a separation takes place which can only increase as it goes. It is necessary to know and understand a child to give him even the part-time attention he does need. Not many parents seem to enjoy their child's company. This is amply supported by their eagerness to find for them some diversion outside of the home. The time is not far past when the dime was handed to the child for the corner movie house as an easy way out. Now it is even easier, a seat in front of the television set and a turn of the knob.

There is a kind of freedom which can be a burden to any individual. And the weight is particularly heavy on the shoul-ders of a child. We have seen that limitations can be felt as support rather than restraint, if thoughtfully planned. Free-dom in excess presents the young child with many choices which he is unprepared to make. He may well mask his anxiety under the cover of a deceptively aggressive behavior. There can be no doubt that children need rules to limit them. This is well demonstrated in an experiment made by Susan Isaacs in the early years of progressive education.[12] Children of nursery school age were assembled in a mode of group life which did not include any rules. Children responded promptly by formulating rules of their own with a keen intuition that rules are necessary for group living. Freedom, to carry its whole meaning, presupposes a grasp of all choices and the inner strength to choose. We all have been reminded of the child suffering from the excessive freedom of progressive education in its early stages. "Do I have to do what I want to?" This is where freedom become a burden. In the same way a child today can have a day so thickly scheduled with opportunities for freedom that he may resent the tediousness of these opportunities. It is the children, and they are many, who have not learned the meaning of freedom, who moan before unscheduled minutes, "I'm bored. What shall I do next?"

Retaining our individual ability to choose and to reason enables us to bind the threads of our life together and to stand as strong individuals. Weak as separates, young people starting off in marriage cannot very well be expected to make wise choices toward their life in common. They have the freedom to build their life together as they wish, only if they have been able to comprehend all the choices.

It is easy to lose track of oneself in the mass of ready-made ideas and waves of emotional stimuli which are proffered at us. Relieved of the necessity and privilege of thinking, one can still be provided with formed opinions. Confusion and a feeling of emptiness must follow the adoption of ready-made standards. For these standards vary from day to day, from newspaper to newspaper, from community to community. One decision of one's own, one idea painstakingly thought out and simple as it is, these are worth to the individual all the weighty opinions gleaned from newspaper, radio, television, and magazine.

Family life is bounded and enriched by the limitations of reality, and if children share in family life, joys and frustrations alike, they will be better prepared in later years to build their own families on the same image.

Something has happened to human relations. People move farther and farther apart from one another. They no longer have the time to know each other, to empathize with and understand each other. Inner-generated communication is at a low level. There is a great need for tightening up the family—not to wish it back where it was but to make it again a close group where each member can live with a sense of fulfillment, both as an individual and as a part of the group.

O. Spurgeon English has emphasized the need for closer family communication.

In spite of the increasing speed of our existence, it appears doubtful if we will prosper unless we learn the importance of pausing frequently to come in touch with each other more tenderly and wisely. The family has always been the place for this phenomenon and society has always blessed it. We must be careful not to squander this heritage. It is the common denominator of the best kind of living of the past and the precepts of modern dynamic psychology.[13]

MARRIAGE AND MATURITY

The majority of young people marrying today do so with little and last-minute preparation. This is implied in early marriages. That the divorce courts are full is hardly surprising when we stop to consider marriage and family life in our time. The full load of responsibility falls from the start on the husband and wife, and full maturity is expected from them at the outset. They begin alone, usually asking no help and receiving none from their families. For the large family unit no longer exists. Not only are husband and wife alone, but other stresses are theirs. They must live in a society that has been uprooted from its past and cannot yet find its bearings in the present. It can offer them no guide to a firmly based marriage. Quite the opposite, they must be able to stay fixed in their own beliefs despite the changing standards around them. To the timid objecting of their parents young people are ready with an answer, "So if it doesn't work out we can always get a divorce."

When does sound preparation begin? Certainly not upon engagement. For it must be an emotional preparation well engrained in the individual. This can begin no later than birth, ideally before that with the parents' marriage. And there we must pause, as often the parents' marriage has been an emotional miscarriage.

We are a long way from the solution to this problem. Attempts have been made to help young people, fragmentary attempts which hit at the periphery, not the core. The most obvious of measures aimed at building happier marriages is the profession of marriage counseling, a discipline still in its infancy. Although counselors are recruited from the ranks of obstetricians, psychologists, social workers, educators, ministers, and psychiatrists, no special training is required. Requirements for its practice not yet clearly defined, it is a matter of chance that his own personality and education will fit him for the task, not to mention the self-appointed, untrained, or worse, a not altogether negligible quantum. Probably a limited number of marriage counselors have the understanding and wisdom to cope effectively with the problems that affront them daily. Some clinics have done excellent work. The Marriage Consultation Center of the Community Church in New York, founded by Dr. Abraham Stone, stands high among these.

But marriage counseling usually comes late. Its services are sought by most in an attempt to save a floundering marriage, as is frequently noted in the history of children who have come from families split by legal or emotional divorce. Counseling would fulfill its task, if it were ambitious enough to include earlier years. But then it would have to reach out into the education of children, and thus could become an integral part of marriage preparation.

When young people decide to marry they often consult no one. If they do ask advice, it is most frequently from their family doctor. "We can only afford to have two children," they may explain. Or it may be that they want to wait several years before having children. This problem being solved, that they ask no more advice is indicative. Even if qualified to do so, the doctor may hesitate to give more general counsel. If he does offer suggestions, they will of necessity be casual.

Ministers are perhaps in a better position than marriage counselors to advise young people in search of help. Many ministers have enlarged the activities of their church to include not only formal religious matters but also the family and social life of their parishioners. Rather, they are gradually recapturing a function which in the past was taken for granted. There are nursery schools for the youngest. And when they grow older there will be picnics and hikes and dances. In this way a minister knows his congregation every day, not only in their Sunday best.

The case of one minister, typical of many, comes to mind. He wanted to know the members of his church well. And to do so he became familiar with psychology in its healthy and morbid aspects, attending lectures and seminars. His knowledge of the Bible and his belief in the ethical principles within its pages led him to put these principles into the practice of his life and his dealings with others. He was wise enough to know that his Sunday sermon was only a forerunner to his work. Scientific knowledge enriched his religious training. He used the two woven together to help his parishioners in their family problems.

He knew when to urge gently an overprotective mother to let up on her son. He could suggest that the shy little girl be given extra encouragement by her family. And when young people came to him with the news that they were to be married, he knew them so well he could offer advice and constructive suggestions toward their happiness together.

Actually, the substance of marriage counseling lies ahead. For every boy and girl who receive any guidance at all, a vast number plunge into marriage with their eyes shut. Under such conditions the plunge is almost bound to be icy, for the realities of life are not easy to face unprepared. The adjustment of one person to another is a delicate one in all situations, let alone in one where the sharing and intimacy can offer cause for stress and friction. It takes time, and it takes maturity to make it successful. This reality should be recognized before marriage. If not, what can marriage be but disillusionment? The rate of divorce has an answer to this question.

Marriage counseling can be helpful. But if it is alone it comes too late. Its radius is insufficient of itself. The ground must be prepared by an emotionally robust childhood. Parents who are happily married will give this to their children. Any last-minute advice offered by minister, doctor, counselor or parent must depend in its final effect on the young person's emotional development from the earliest years on.

But surely, some would reason, certain aspects of preparation for marriage had better be postponed until just before the wedding. And sex education is usually the argument first on their list. A glance into the issue will show that an acceptance of sex begins in the home, not with books, but with mature and sexually adjusted parents.

It is not, as many would have it, a question of whether or not to let a child know about sex, for at some stage every child is faced with this information, and to a much greater extent misinformation. The opportunities for gathering it are many. If we were to keep this aspect of life a closed book to children, they would have to be sheltered from radio, television, movies, newspapers, and the company of their friends. And even then they would have some perception of their parents' marital relations, with the coloring dependent upon the nature of these relations.

It is with a totally unrealistic view that parents protest the sex education offered by schools. Such education is probably the safest the child has had, if he has not already received it in the family. Information offered by schools can only act as a corrective to the distorted pictures built upon mass programs indiscriminately displayed for any audience, adult or child, not to mention vivid references overheard from older children.

It has been the attempt of schools to offer objective knowledge about sex. In this way they hope to avoid unwanted emotional overtones. With diagrams, movies, and lectures they acquaint children with ungarnished fact. Thus they hope that the child may be spared the unwholesome and frightening interpretations.

Public schools have set a difficult task for themselves. They are trying to educate a large and varied group of children on a subject that is best passed on individually. Information and the mode of presentation must be regulated in terms of the child's current knowledge and emotional attitude. The question period will be of little value for the timid child. And one who has lived a sheltered existence hardly needs the same information as the child who has picked up more or less explicit terminology from city streets.

We have said that the public school's view is unrealistic when they aim at objectivity. Can there be an objective lecture given? It must in some way be colored by the teacher's

289

attitude, her own conflicts, small or great, as well as the attitudes of her pupils. Children can immediately discern embarrassment masked in scientific objectivity. Sex is part of a broader human relationship. No human relationship can be explained merely by objective scientific analysis. The biological story is but half the story and, if anything, the less important half. The child psychiatrist is familiar with the youngster who can reel off all the biological details and yet have not absorbed the emotional impact to the extent of complete block.

The teacher's attitude can make the lecture helpful or it can make it meaningless and even harmful. But more important is the individual student's own feelings on the subject. Among the students there will be varying degrees of understanding, confusion, fear, and resentment. And each child should be individually understood, before an explanation of sex can meet its full purpose.

In an age now past many children had an immediate opportunity to become acquainted with the phenomenon of birth. In the country they saw the mare ready to foal, they saw the newborn calf take its first wobbly step by its mother's side, not to mention rabbits, cats, dogs, and others of the animal world. There was no shroud of mystery to impart a sense of taboo. Now, schools in industrial areas are trying to restore to children something of this closeness to nature. They have nature-study classes where third and fourth graders keep guinea pigs and hamsters at school, feeding and caring for them. Nature camps are also plentiful.

But this is not enough. The substitute is only a partial answer. On the farm, birth was a natural event, a part of the child's life. The bull was pastured with the cows, and in the spring calves were born. Little Benjie, the child of "Love Is Enough" in *Children of Divorce*,[14] spontaneously announced that a calf had just been born. Little wonder to him, even if he was not acquainted with procreation taboos between unrelated species. The sexes were appropriate. The horse, a male, and the cow had been under the tree in the field long enough. And now there was their child. For rural children the cycle of new life follows the turning of the seasons; it is a regular and unquestioned process. And the birth of a baby brother or sister seems just as natural. The mother wasn't taken away to a hospital, but stayed in her own room at home. And there the child could see the baby as soon as he was born.

Despite all attempts at substitution, this natural climate for a child's growth cannot be recaptured. In the city, natural processes pass unnoticed. Even the seasons are of minor importance. There is no sowing, no harvesting. Once a child could feel secure in the recurring round of natural events. Now that source of security has vanished. School and no school is more likely to be the cycle for the city child.

Schools cannot make up the loss. Theirs is a part-time job, and it is taken up late. They can give only a small amount of attention to the child individually, and at best on the biological end of the story. Of necessity they work in partial blindness, since they cannot visualize each child in his home. It is there, in the home, that the most important preparation must be made.

An emotional acceptance of sex is of greater importance than a scientific understanding. And it must come first. Before the school presents charts and lectures on conception and birth, the child should have been able to absorb the emotional impact of a subject alive all about him—then and only then can he profit from a knowledge of its biological aspects.

The total aim of sex education is to foster the child's emotional growth as a preparation for a happy adult life. This is not within the compass of the school's teachings. For, the focus of a child's emotional life is his family. It may either provide an atmosphere of warmth and love which will head him on toward acceptance, or his parents' tension and unhappiness—left unsaid or exploding in scenes—may permeate with anxiety the child's approach to sex. The factual sex information that parents pass on to their children counts much less than the emotional overtones. All too often their own troubled feelings are the sum total of those overtones. "My wife is frigid and I have my work," says the father of a twelve-year-old girl, whose severe anxiety has created a multiplicity of somatic symptoms. The father in his concise statement presents the marital problem as non-existent. The sexual discontent is shut out, water tight, from the child. So both parents feel assured. The father drives himself to work to the edge of tolerance, and his wife's own sexual urges can be disregarded, since satisfaction is not possible. But any psychiatrist knows, and this is the case here, that through the years the child has reacted with gradually increasing intolerable anxiety to the parents' sexual conflict.

The task of providing their children with adequate information on sex looms for many parents as an uneasy enterprise if not a frightening ordeal. If their own sexual life has been entangled with frustration and inhibition, they may compensate with an exaggerated license. This is an ineffectual way of cancelling their own uneasiness. Their children are made to live in a home where restrictions have been discarded, where there is no privacy in the bathroom, where nudism is almost enforced. Yet these same parents too pointedly shy from demonstrations of affection for one another.

Other parents "shelter" their children and spare themselves embarrassment, so they think, by ignoring the subject, clinging to the hope that their children will pick up the needed information from some source or other. The silent pall that hangs over the matter is guarantee that their children will not ask questions. These are the same parents who are convinced that their child was "not interested in those things. . . . He never asked questions . . . ," a statement frequently heard by the psychiatrist in the course of history-taking.

These solutions are not solutions, for they disregard reality. It is unrealistic to create for a child a topsy-turvy world where people parade naked, for he will never live in such a world. It is equally unrealistic to expect a child to develop healthy attitudes toward the unmentionable. His parents' own inner feelings will most strongly influence his attitudes. Let there be no doubt about it, to the child's antennae there are no hidden feelings.

Nor is there reality in the suggestion that we resume a rural life where our children can live in close contact with nature and its biological offerings. Children today are born in antiseptic hospitals, kept in large nurseries, and then brought home to city apartments. The infant begins his life remote from his parents, brothers and sisters. In the face of dense agglomeration of large cities today the inevitability of this state of affairs would seem apparent. However, in small ways this is being changed through the rooming-in plan which affords closeness between mother and newborn infant. To the siblings the birth event remains a detached, far-away experience.

What is it that children need to know about sex? What is it that they should be told? When a child asks his first question, perhaps where he came from or how his little brother arrived, he will not be asking for the totality of biological facts as adults know them. Many parents overwhelm their children with "scientific" information where a few words would suffice. What a young child needs to know, rather, is that sex (even as he is ignorant of the word, he senses the relation) between his parents is a happy thing, and that while it is a private matter, it includes him, for it was through such love that he came into the world. The child is interested primarily in what affects him. His world of necessity, for a number of years begins and ends with himself. This is the natural egocentricity of the young child.

The emotional climate his parents provide is far more important than detailed scientific fact. The child psychiatrist, despite his awareness and his understanding of underlying mechanisms, is again and again impressed with the parallel existence in one child of complete knowledge of biological fact and lack of emotional insight.

To illustrate, Peter, a four-year-old boy of very superior intelligence, the only child of older parents, is seen in the midst of a period of dramatization of the conception and birth phenomena. In his nursery school group many of the children at this particular time are playing out the life drama as each feels it. Peter has a theme of his own, a confused one which is indeed revealing.

His parents come from a highly intellectual and cultivated social stratum. Their attitudes are very proper and rather prudish with an admixture of overly liberal concepts about child education. They have been at great pains to give him early all the biological knowledge they felt necessary. How has Peter absorbed this knowledge? In his play he dramatizes as follows: he is the father and he is going to "make a baby." To this effect he has seed in his bags which he is going to distribute (sowing) here and there (pointing in space rather vaguely). If the destination of the seeds is somewhat indefinite and multiple, their origin is well focused. They come from South America, where they were bought and put in little bags. When the seeds are connected with eggs (origin and nature not determined) a baby will begin to grow. Interspersed through the fantasy are words of anatomical description which are irrelevant to the fantasy and, as he gives them, unrelated to one another (vagina, ovary, tubes, etc.). Wherefrom could such confusion arise in a very bright boy who has also an amazing fund of knowledge in various areas such as geography, history, etc., and who has been, as his mother assures us, "told everything about it"?

We are impressed with the fact that Peter has learned a great many biological details but has been unable to absorb them and make them part of his apprehension of the birth concept. In passing, the South American element is traced to the contemporaneous return of a favorite relative from South America with many tales of strange flowers and artificial pollenization. This much for the play fantasy. On the other hand, we know that Peter giggles a great deal at the mention of bathroom terminology popular with the nursery school child, lifts girls' skirts, peeps at his parents' bedroom more than the average child of his age, and generally reveals an intense curiosity about sex. Needless to say, the plethora of biological details has not satisfied his curiosity. The emotional climate of his home has not been conducive to this satisfaction.

Words are hardly necessary to tell a child that his parents are happy in that he is part of their love. If he feels the joy and warmth they radiate as lovers and as parents, questions on sex will cause him little anxiety. Even before he asks questions he will have an answer in the emotional climate of his home.

If, however, he senses discord between his parents, if he feels their tension and frustration with each other, his attitude toward sex will be confused and full of anxiety. It cannot be associated with his parents' love for each other or for him. It follows that parents should look into their marital conflicts for their children's sake, if not for their own, for it is in those conflicts that later difficulties in adulthood and marriage can be traced.

Parents who find their marital life unrewarding need not feel alone. Medical reports show that many couples in America today fail to enjoy a satisfactory sex life. Rather than continue in their plight these couples might look into its causes and get help in solving it. One small instance: if they understand the hidden hostility and frustration that lie behind their sudden angry outbursts toward their marriage partner or children, that anger will lose some of its intensity. And, remote as it may seem to them, it should now be evident that even if biological facts can be learned in a few schema, sex education cannot be dispensed a few days before the marriage ceremony, and that preparation for marriage is not a specific small compartment of knowledge. A child's real preparation for marriage begins with his parents' own marriage.

Marriage today would be founded upon love, sometimes love at the exclusion of all other considerations. It was not so in the past. As we have seen, boys and girls were very early trained in the practical aspects of womanhood and manhood, because it was then thought that in the wake of these achievements love would come. Tortuous as the road may have been, sometimes it did. In the home the girl learned to be a homemaker and a mother. And the boy grew up knowing that he must later take on full responsibilities. It is true that something very important was lacking in this home instruction, for the ideal of love did not enter.

Limited and blind as it was, this training had something which we no longer offer children today, a definite standard of conduct, a clear knowledge of the roles of man and woman, and an attempt at forming personalities for this role. Children then knew the exigencies of marriage before they were married; they knew the demands that would be made upon them. That sex references were not included is transparent in Victorian memoirs. They accepted these demands for they learned them early. The girl knew the satisfaction of caring for a home and family. Her position was secure. She knew the skills necessary for her job.

And so did the boy know his responsibility, knew that he would have to be the home builder. He also knew that his position as head of the family was a dignified one of which he was justifiably proud.

Today the family has fallen into some confusion. The mother is part-bread-winner, the father is part-housekeeper. And neither knows exactly what is expected of him or her. The wife, officially or in more subtle ways, may have the position of head of the family with her husband's consequent lack of dignity.

One reason for the break-down of the family may be the distorted importance the individual has taken on in society today, an importance which is not without its share of conflict owing to the parallel drive to conform. The individual comes first, before community, before family, but at the same time is expected to meet heavy demands from the social group. Women often resent or ignore the responsibility of devoting themselves to their families. Men may not experience the full impact of their obligation to support their families. Both men and women are looking for something else, for position, for wealth, for all the acquisitions that are so important in our material age.

Their concept of responsibility has been absorbed by their children. Little wonder is it that we hear the reports from all sides. Children have lost respect and consideration for others. Similarly, they have lost respect for the property of others. Parents may well think that ethics is a special department of teaching with which they will in time deal adequately. Here, as in all cases, however, what they are, not what they teach, will be the touch-stone of their accomplishment. A young matron, respected in her community, and who can be considered by general standards as honest and ethical, gloats at having "put something over" on her landlord. The landlord pays for the electricity and she for the gas. Very pleased with herself, she announces to a friend that having recently installed an electric stove, unbeknownst to her landlord, she now saves ten dollars a month. Her two-year-old little boy is present. He has stopped rolling his small car back and forth and looks at his mother with intense curiosity. He has not understood the mathematics nor the ethics involved, but he has heard the change in the voice, he has seen the gleam in his mother's eyes and the remolding of her facial expression. He has registered a picture—special, different from his other well-known pictures of his mother—a picture which is to re-appear in similar subtly shrewd situations where the mother unguardedly will again reveal her cleverness. In later years when his mother will attempt to educate him on what is right and wrong, it is not so much the words she will proffer that he will hear, but rather the accumulated emotional impact of her shrewdness.

This is one small situation involving one individual. But the disregard of other people's rights is not so localized. A school teacher testifies that in her thirty years in city schools she has seen children change from responsible to generally careless, if not outright destructive. In the past a child who had torn a school book would be frightened of the conse-quences in and out of himself. Today books are torn, cut, marked, and lost. And, knowing that there are more where they came from, children, not having been early impressed with a sense of responsibility, continue in their destruction.

Part of the story of vandalism is told in the figures given by the Park Commissioner of New York City. He reported that during one recent year children under sixteen caused damage to the city for the specific amount of $204,361. This is only city property. Add to it slashed tires, carved up walls, broken windows, and other by-products of children's amusements.

The most obvious explanation for this behavior on the part of children would be poverty and slum life. It is natural to imagine that these children are underprivileged and looking for redress. Statistics on delinquency in slum areas seem to bear this out. But that is not always the case. Vandals come from all economic levels. Suburbanites will testify to this. They have many stories to tell of neighborhood children from "good" backgrounds who break into houses, smash win-dows, steal, all in search of diversion. The reader will recall the account of house breaking and vandalism in an abandoned house in Westchester county.

Rural districts are not left out in the story of vandalism. In a small agricultural community an elderly couple—the man retired on a small pension from his life work with a large industrial organization—have managed in recent years and by dint of self-deprivation to accumulate enough cash for that one Florida vacation they must have before they die. In a happy mood they go. It is not long before their house is spotted as unoccupied. Two boys, under fifteen, see adventure in that, for the weak inner structure and idleness call for adventure. At dusk they enter the house, an elaborate process, since the old people have been cautious. There is not much of value in this house. Disappointment follows the thorough but futile search for valuables.

Frustrated, as a wilful four-year-old would be who has not been heeded in his excessive demands, the two boys have a tantrum, a tantrum expensive to the owners of this house: slashing draperies, cutting up rugs, hammering the furniture to bits. This brings up the cost of damage to a minimal thousand dollars, an extravagant sum for the old people. Advisedly, the behavior of these teen-agers has been compared to the tantrum of earlier years. Indeed, delinquency and vandalism, protean in their manifestations, have a common denominator, a poorly developed ego. In this instance the original motivation, i.e., acquiring valuables, is clear, and while unjustifiable, can be understood. But sheer wanton destruction, perhaps even more frequently encountered, offers no immediately understandable motivation outside of impulses. An understanding of the nature of these impulses would require volumes of behavior analysis, and quite a few of these have been written.

In the following picture, drawn from another rural community, we find the sheer wanton destruction without apparent motivation which is so general in the countryside but does not, for that matter exclude urban communities. A property in the process of being transferred to a new owner is, for a brief period, without occupants. Although liberally sprinkled along its boundaries with posters that bear the stamp of the police department authority in addition to the more negligible one of the owner, it naturally becomes a playground for the local teen-agers. Without ammunition, ideas for games would run short. So along come the guns. At a little distance from the main house stands a barn with some twelve windows, an irresistible target in the sunlight. Picnic fashion, beer has also been brought in generous quantity. It is a matter of weeks before the barn displays gaping holes in place of window panes. Beer bottles come in handy too, when ammunition runs out.

The process of destruction goes on at a slower pace for the log cabin which also stands nearby. Out goes the bed from the loft, piece by piece, on what would seem to be a well-organized plan. The walls, the floors, the roof are pulled apart and thrown about. The tide of destruction reaches the dismantling of the beautiful stone fireplace. It takes plenty of energy and even a crowbar to pull the flue out, but that also is accomplished. The owner had watched helplessly the dissolution of his property. The police had been co-operative but powerless. Now, something must be done about the physical damage. A contractor was called in to assess the cost of repair. He was not overly concerned, nor was he surprised. While discussing the damage with the owner, he offered a neat explanation, "Boys will be boys." Optimistically he suggested a practical way of protecting the property from future damage. "Invite them in and give them a party. . . . Cake and soda pop will do. . . . They will leave your place alone."

Thus the solution has been reached by one man, the "party bribe." Such are the solutions offered by many parents in coping with their children's behavior. Unable to discipline them, they hope to keep them in line with a system of rewards and bonuses.

The destructive drive is native. It belongs to an early stage of normal development. It does not label a child as "bad." But as the years go by it must be controlled and sublimated into socially acceptable outlets. It is the parents' job patiently to help their children to control their impulses, to direct them into competitive sports, constructive hobbies, etc., to help them develop an awareness of other people's rights alongside their own.

Patience is for many too hard a task. A man may be very successful at slowly training his dog in the field, quietly and patiently teaching him to point and retrieve. But the same man is helpless when it comes to disciplining his son. He finds it easier to let the boy go his own way. Not until the latter does something particularly antisocial or gets into trouble outside of the home does he attempt discipline by angry shouting and severe punishment.

299

Perhaps the analogy between the training of a dog and of a child will shock some. But the analogy remains just the same. An untrained child can be more distressing to his parents than an untrained dog. And unfortunate it is that he is seen more frequently.

The comparison breaks down. For while animal pets respond to love (like children they show an uncanny sureness of perception of man's true feelings), they can be trained without it. Not so a child. A child needs love and understanding, not domination or abandonment to his instinctual impulse. Some parents, unable to give such understanding to their children, substitute either rigid discipline or unlimited freedom, or alternate one with the other as their mood dictates.

Trouble starts early for the child of such parents. Undisciplined, he will have a hard time adjusting to the give and take of friendship and to the demands of education. Can we see him as a happy adult? Without a sound basis to cope with reality will he be able to accept frustrations?

Vandalism, a recall of the fifth century Teutons who devastated Gaul and Rome, is a very general phenomenon of our times. It does not, as the dictionary definition would have it, mean only the willful destruction of what is beautiful and artistic. Mismotivated as the Vandals might have been, they were intent on destroying the artistic achievements of civilizations they abhorred. The wanton destruction which is usually referred to as vandalism is something other. It is an expression of the immaturity of those who abandon themselves to it. It is the deed of children who have not known restraint, who have not learned the long, slow lesson of self-discipline. These are the children who do not accept the bounds of reality. For reality is a hard taskmaster.

Not long ago, hoping to undo what were considered extremes in the disciplining of children, psychiatrists suggested a certain leniency in child training. Many parents snatched at this advice and used as much of it as suited their own needs. That is, they accepted the leniency and by-passed the necessary restrictions. Without shading, the easier way out becomes in the end the hardest of all. They gave their children free scope for venting their aggressions. With this directive they could feel that their children were being given a chance to express themselves, while they were spared the task of guiding them from instant to instant. A general tendency that: easy, easier, the easiest. A valuable movement in child study thus degenerated in many circles to a facile, but in the end harmful, approach to children and no relief to their parents.

Much that children learn is by "imitation" of adults (actually, identification with them). By taking the lead from their parents little girls will want to develop the attributes of femininity, while boys will emulate the masculine characteristics of their fathers. That, at least, is the hoped-for pattern.

What is it that boys learn from their fathers today? Why is it that they, rather than girls, so generally engage in destructive practices? Is such practice set before them as an example of masculinity?

In a subtle way it is. Ours is a woman-dominated society. Women today are assumed to have many virtues. This idealization of women is typically American. Writers from other countries have repeatedly recorded this observation. The British anthropologist Geoffrey Gorer has commented at length on this phenomenon.[15] One small facet of it is evident in our schools. Children almost invariably receive their ethical training from women. Seldom teaching elementary or junior high school, men are too often found in senior high school (where their influence anyway would carry less weight), teaching only a few subjects, mathematics, science, and of course athletics. Even before attending school, children's ethical training is feminine, from their mothers and their nurses.

The "virtuous" man is frequently a butt of jokes. He is thought to be namby-pamby. To get along in our competitive world the man is expected to be smart, aggressive, ruthless, if necessary. He is commended for "putting something over" on the other fellow. The story of many a successful business is given in just these terms, barely disguised.

If men are scorned for the "soft" qualities of virtue, women on the other hand are extolled for the possession of these. The boy grows up seeing his mother as an epitome of all that is good. In his mind she is a creature quite above the masculine world. And when he looks for a girl to marry, he looks for what he takes for granted in his mother. When she proves only human, his dream is painfully shattered.

301

But the boy must assert his masculinity and in so doing feels called upon to defy the woman-made rules. This has a glamour of its own. Everyone is prone to like the aggressive, "bad boy." Even his mother finds him more attractive than her less defiant, more passive son—even if she is, as often the case, excessively attached to the latter. This bad boy becomes the hero of movies, while the gentle, well-mannered boy is labelled a sissy.

The father has little part in the boy's early moral training. Yet a boy will tend to reject the ideals his mother represents, for those ideals will, for him, be associated with the feminine world. Only from his father's example could he feel that goodness and manliness are not antonymous. How can fathers give their sons such an example, if society demands other values?

Too many parents are prone to trust to the future to reform their young hellion into a respectable citizen. At his first brush with the law they are quick to say, "He's learning the hard way." Can one learn so fast and make a turn-about from one's already-stamped personality? Parents comfort themselves with the belief that their son is going through an aggressive-destructive stage which he will outgrow. The transformation will come at seventeen or nineteen or twenty-one. Then it is hoped that the boy will suddenly become a man. Perhaps the army will do the trick, or perhaps marriage and a family, the "growing-out-of-it magic."

Once in a while we do see a boy settle down to the responsibilities of adult living after a stint in the army or upon getting married and starting a family. But can these last-minute measures really change an emotionally immature person into a stable and responsible individual? Can a few months make up for many lost years?

The frustrated, destructive, irresponsible child does not disappear. He remains more or less successfully hidden through the years, perhaps known only to his wife and children. They know him through his daily irritability, his tantrums of temper, his moods. And perhaps the psychiatric clinic will know him too, for he may emerge as an individual emotionally disturbed in various degrees.

Sometimes immaturity, concealed successfully for a time,

makes known its presence in a sudden explosion. Thus recorded by a daily paper, here is a case.

The Vice President of the —— Bank and Trust Company, a man prominent in civic affairs and highly trusted by his employers, was arrested here tonight on a charge of embezzling $400,000 of the bank's funds.

—— is married and has three children . . . a mild mannered man known in the community for his pleasing personality . . . fifty years old . . . long prominent in community affairs . . . a warden and Sunday School teacher at —— Church and chairman of the church's trust fund committee, local director of the American Red Cross, chairman of the committee of the Boy Scout fund raising campaign, chairman of the Community Chest Fund.

Mayor ——, informed of the arrest, said, "I am amazed and stunned." Rev. ——, pastor of —— Church, said, "The news knocked the legs out from under me. I can't believe it."

—— is believed to have used the money to gamble in the stock market. His salary as bank Vice President is $8,500 a year.

And this story is by no means unique. We have all read it in its more spectacular form, in subtler shadings, and more frequently, in psychiatric records. For, the child who has not gradually learned the disciplines and restraints of reality remains a child, however successful and highly developed he appears. The business man may wonder why his little girl is not learning self-control. He would be the last to realize that his behavior is no different. He has, of course, no insight into his own immaturity. Responsibility can be a crippling burden, if it falls upon a man who remains emotionally a child. Our records of suicides, broken marriages, mental illness, and tonnage of sedatives, laxatives, and tranquilizers used will attest to that.

When exactly does the child start becoming an adult? At what point in his life must we turn over to him adult responsibilities? There is, of course, no exact time. The child begins his growth toward adulthood from the very time of his birth. This is an aphorism, but it needs to be reiterated. It is not long before he must get acquainted with the inescapable disciplines.

Every age has its limitations, its rules, its responsibilities. Many parents fail to realize this. They wait until their son or daughter has grown to adult size. And then, only then, do they demand that he or she show a sense of responsibility. With the right to drink and vote conferred upon him, the child is expected to about-face into a man.

I have considered the more general maturing of the individual as the basic preparation for a successful marriage. The last step to marriage is the choice of a marriage partner. But this decision, as all others, was determined many years before marriage was even thought of. The parents' marriage, the years of childhood, these go into his choice of whom to marry. The young person's attitude toward his or her parents, his attitude toward his home, the love he has or has not received and given during childhood, these and many other factors go into his decision to get married and the very choice of a partner.

How can he, or she, be best prepared to make this choice? What help can he get and from whom when he is planning for marriage? How can a girl be guided in deciding on her future husband? In years past the success of a marriage depended largely on its financial stability and the assuming of well-defined responsibilities—a rigid frame of reference. The girl's father spoke with the young man on his ability to support his daughter. We do not look for financial stability to such a definite extent now, in part because this has become a transitory and somewhat elusive quantity in our time. Fluctuations of success and failure have become part of the modern economic pattern, and the reverberations on the individual can easily be discerned.

What sound base is there for marriage grounded on romance without the support of economic stability? Today the most important thing we can look for is emotional stability. A young man can provide his home with a sound emotional atmosphere, a stability which will stand through success or failure, only if he is himself emotionally mature. This stability is not as easy to measure as a bank balance.

It is true that a harmonious home will bring about adjustment of the children in it. But is a home unbroken by divorce necessarily a harmonious home? The choice of marriage partners on a neurotic basis is well known to the psychiatrist. One of the most destructive homes ever known to the writer was one in which the sado-masochistic relation between the parents was, one might say, airtight. There was no escape from the reciprocal tyranny of these parents. From the start and on the eve of their marriage they were "perfect for each other," so the amateur psychologist had formed his opinion after independent testing of the young people by the bridegroom.

It is hardly necessary to point out again that devastating conflicts exist, not only in homes already broken by divorce, but in those homes where divorce is the only step that has not yet been taken in the estrangement of man and wife. While no brief need be held for divorce, it may in the long run be helpful to the child, if it makes him free of an atmosphere of hatred and conflict. And, if his parents can both give him the necessary assurance of their love during and after their divorce, he may be well on his way to a normal adult and married life despite the early loss.

Marriage is all too often entered to satisfy a short-lived sexual attraction, a passion which may be romantic but not often realistic. The only protection a young person can have against such infatuation is the background of his own family life as a maturing experience, the background of a love shared in the give and take of daily living. This love, experienced through childhood and adolescence, will not admit of the substitution of romantic love.

That is not to say that romantic love does not play a very important part as the basis for a happy marriage. Romantic love includes sexual love, a focal point in the marriage relationship. Although a marriage cannot stand firm on sexual attraction and satisfaction alone, it can hardly be a rich and full marriage without it. Sexual love enriched by affection and understanding is a most necessary part of a successful marriage.

Just as sexual love alone can play havoc when it instigates marriage, so can love based solely on romance. For then, the idealized partner must suddenly come down to earth and play the role of father or mother, provider or homemaker. Then the real person must come to the fore, the substance behind the shadow. If a young person has known a happy family life, sharing both happiness and sorrow, partaking in work as well as play, the realities of marriage will then be its deepest satisfactions. This is the mature person. Love and affection received early have enabled the child to move into progressive forms of the capacity to love, extending now beyond members of the family. Such a person will instinctively look for a marriage partner who shows similar maturity. For them not a marriage in which neurotic seeks neurotic with immaturities and distorted urges at play in a war of the sexes. For them marriage is not viewed as a short-time affair with divorce easily available. "If it doesn't work out we can always divorce," says many a young aspirant to marriage today, an echo we are familiar with.

Many parents find it difficult to include their children in family life, troubles and all. This is a matter of deeper communication than the scant superficial chatter with one ear cocked to the television program. Fearing to subject their children to worry, thinking in terms of an illusory bliss based on total removal of disappointment, parents exclude their children. Financial difficulties are discussed behind closed doors, while the children know only the uneasiness they sense in the air. Sickness may occur, but they are spared the concerns attached. Adults, because of their own immaturities, meet the painful realities of life with a disproportionate degree of anxiety or panic. The multiplicity of agencies and devices to insure modern man against uncertainty attest to this: social security, accident or illness insurance, life insurance, unemployment benefits, etc. We make a fetish of easy living, and thus hardships, great and small, are not tolerated with equanimity. This is the "softness" that comes out so glaringly at times of great stress, such as war conscription or economic depression. It has been commented upon by many psychiatrists.

From their own panic parents attempt to protect their children. But children have antennae of their own. The inarticulate voice of the unknown is more threatening to them than any reality, however painful. Suppose that parents succeed in raising a child in a fool's paradise, totally carefree. Suppose that child has never had to cope with frustrations, these having been systematically eased off by well-intentioned parents;

306

suppose he has never shared in the work of the family group. This child will grow up and eventually be labelled "adult" by the law. He will suddenly be faced with a drama for which there has been no rehearsal. Each small difficulty will rise before his eyes as a crisis. His parents will have passed on to him an inheritance of insecurity and fear. In this sense can the meaning of heredity, strictly applying to characteristics passed on through the genes, be stretched to include the passing on from one generation to the next of near intangibles.

Marriage, in one of its facets, and not one of the least meaningful, is made up of the daily sharing of joys and griefs. A young person unacquainted with a hard core of realities is not ready to look for a husband or wife. For he cannot apprehend the meaning of marriage. He has not known in his family the love that grows from sharing emotional experiences. The groundwork for a happy marriage is prepared many years before the couple have met. No last-minute measures, no cramming can substitute.

The news of a marriage is greeted with automatic approval. The unmarried girl is pitied. We have all seen the concern of parents whose children have grown to the age of twenty-five and remain unmarried. A sense of failure hovers about these young people. Society nods its approval at marriage. It looks askance at those who remain single.

Rare are the young people who would dare to admit, even to themselves, that they would prefer to remain single, that they long neither for marriage nor for children. Very few would even dare to wait until they felt ready for marriage, perhaps years after the socially recognized standard.

It is true that for the majority of men and women marriage is the most natural and satisfying way to achieve love and companionship. And for most of these, children provide self-fulfillment. This being granted, should we not raise the question of whether some could not, single, live just as happy and just as full a life? Could they not find achievement and joy in their work and self-giving in forms other than married love? Others are happily married without children, whether they had so planned or not. They achieve a full life in each other and in their work. Why is it that we insist on the one form of fulfillment for every person?

Convention has powerful forces on its side. Its standards enable people to live together in community life with the greatest ease possible. Therefore, convention is important, but it must be interpreted for each individual. Marriage is the conventional way of adult life. Is it the only way? Many young people follow it simply in order to escape being "different." Passing reference can be made to the eldest daughter of eleven children in the Lewis family of *Children of Divorce*, where a twelfth child, Benjie, was adopted. Unmarried—and in the general mind sacrificed to the younger brood—she radiates nevertheless with happiness and a sense of fulfillment. Her lot as she feels it or as others can judge of it does not seem to have been in any way less happy than the rest of the family.

The "spinster" receives more pity than she needs in our society. We tend to look upon her as someone who was not able to get married. Seldom do we speculate that she might have preferred to remain single and have found much happiness in her life. We have only to recall one of the maiden aunts of the recent past who enjoyed family life to the full, loving and loved by nieces and nephews, to know that unmarried life need not turn a woman into a cranky "spinster." These women have dared to choose a life for which they were emotionally suited, instead of trying to fit uncomfortably into society's mold. A trend toward accepting aloneness, as a matter of fact, is reflected in titles such as "Live Alone and Like It."

Elaborate statistics tell us that there is a predominance of unmarried people among the population of mental hospitals. An independent thinker, familiar with the statistics, astutely commented with a quip, which for all its facetiousness is worth a second thought. "Sure, the others (the married ones) are busy keeping the intake line at a good pace." When we think of neurotic marriages and their frequency, the quip takes on substance.

With all our talk about the individual today why is he so hard to find? Very few people have the courage to differ from their fellows. Children show their natural need to conform in where their family stands, what they should have that others already possess, how they should behave to fit, etc. They form gangs and clubs. But, instead of growing out of their childhood conformity, they seem to try harder for it as they grow older.

Marriage for some will be another stop in conformity, with readiness for it not given a hearing. It will mean a race to keep up with the neighbors, a race to have all the material signs of prosperity, at least one car, possibly two television sets, a membership in "The Club." The children of such a marriage will be measured and compared with the ones next door. Their privileges and restrictions will be set by those accepted in the group. Their grades in school will also be measured against the same standard. The members of such a family have forsaken the lost art of thinking for themselves.

Today particularly, the individual needs emotional strength. The very solidarity and invulnerability of the group depends on the ego strength of the individuals integrated in this group. If husband and wife do not make a success of their marriage, there will be no one else to hold their family together. If they suffer the tension and hostility of an emotional divorce, their children must suffer with them. Each broken marriage, whether legally or only emotionally broken, marks, each in its own way, the disintegration of family life. The solution of the problem lies with each individual. Only with maturity will his marriage be a healthy and rich experience, his family be a true family, and his children emotionally secure and ready in their own time to make a mature choice.

A PERSPECTIVE ON THE FAMILY

Through the centuries the family unit has always been the cornerstone of society. But the function and the structure of the family has differed widely in time and space. Its role has always been the bearing and raising of children. But other roles held in the past have ceased to belong to it.

In ancient Greece and Rome the family was an agent of the law. It was headed by the father, in whose hands was absolute power over all members, the power of life and death. And one punishment he could enforce was particularly significant. That was expulsion from the family, a punishment suffered only for serious offense. A man or woman without a family lost all rights, all means of livelihood. In the eyes of society he was a complete outcast, his only means of existence were crime and piracy. A woman could live only by prostitution. Death could hardly be a more dread sentence. All or none. An individual, part of the family, or nothing.

In the Bible we find evidence that the family functioned as an economic unit. Marriage was then a matter of business. The bride was given to the boy who could pay the price. Under these conditions Jacob labored for Rachael. For seven years he worked for his prospective father-in-law, only to succeed in winning Leah. Seven more years of toil were demanded of him before he could have the hand of Rachael, the girl he loved. We find it difficult to accept such customs. Our way of thinking is merely a matter of different custom. In Jacob's day love was not expected to motivate marriage and was certainly not sufficient apology for it.

Many primitive tribes in our time function on a similar economic structure. In agricultural communities each family member is essential to the economic well-being of the group. Working together in the fields, each contributes his share, mother and children as well as the men. The marriage of a girl in such a family is an economic loss, it must be compensated for by the bridegroom. It appears logical that he should pay a price for his bride. While her family loses, he gains a money earner.

When divorce separates this man and woman, it is assumed that there is little or no emotional upheaval. On the basis of accepted mores the matter can be handled as an economic one. The bride may be at fault because of barrenness or failure to perform her allotted tasks. Then her family must return the bride price and take her back to live among them. The bride price need not be returned, if similar charges can be made against the husband.

And what of the children of such a marriage? If the family is matriarchal, they remain with the mother in her family. If it is patriarchal, they remain in the father's family. In the latter case they do not suffer the loss of a mother, for there are many mother-substitutes to take over their care. In the large kinship groups the welfare of the children does not depend solely, or even primarily, on the parents. Often the mother means little more to the child than any other woman in the clan. The Samoan infant, for instance, is cared for by the next oldest girl who is able to carry him.

The structure of the family of the past and the family of primitive peoples today was and is multiple, a kinship unit in which grandparents, parents, uncles and aunts and cousins live, if not together, at least very close to one another. It is a firmly rooted group in which every member has a secure place, in which responsibility is shared by all and burdens no one individual excessively. It is a family which can absorb comfortably the child without parents, the woman without a husband, a family offering stability and a sense of belonging.

But the passing centuries have brought changes. Further-

311

more, these changes have been revolutionary in our time. Function and structure have altered. Its function now is the bearing and raising of children. Its structure has dwindled down to father and mother and, on the average, one or two children. All responsibility falls on the two adult members of the family. Upon their success as parents lies the future of their children.

The change in Europe began not very long before our own time. It came as the population grew and the land was filled up. There was no longer room for the large family to live on the land of their ancestors. The eldest son became heir to all, the younger were expected to go out into business and make their own livelihood. It was with these changes that the custom arose of providing the daughters of the family with marriage portions so that they might win husbands, for they were no longer an economic asset but rather a liability. The family group gradually began to break down.

The Industrial Revolution increased this process of disintegration. With its onset, whole communities were uprooted. Industry destroyed much of rural living. Men had to go wherever they could find work, separating from their parents, taking their wives and children with them. They turned to the cities, sometimes travelling so far that there was no possibility of visiting the families they had left behind. The change that had been gradually taking place gathered impetus. Our present family structure emerged, the small unit of parents and children, dependent only on one another. And the functions of the family were reduced primarily to that of child rearing.

From the revolutionary thinking of the eighteenth century and from the machine age of the nineteenth there came political and philosophic changes as well. Man as an individual gained importance. His rights were proclaimed, the political right to have a voice in his government, the economic right to undertake work of his own choice and to make his own living. Similarly, his church was his own choice. And marriage became a matter for individual decision. In this climate of individuality did democracy emerge.

With the emphasis on the individual, romantic love became a part of marriage. It was soon to be the socially accepted reason for choosing a mate. And when not actually the motivating force for marriage, it was likely, nevertheless, to coalesce with the true motivation. Economic considerations had once been an honorable incentive to marry. Now a boy might still marry for money, but he usually didn't admit it, even to himself. A girl might marry for social position, but love alone was avowed.

We thus regard what is merely a custom as a basic principle. Marriage without love in the front line seems somehow shameful to us today. But we forget that there were solid values in the marriage of times past. Families then had a stability and a security that we lack today.

Change took place slowly in Europe but was abrupt in America. People sought the colonies as an escape from the controls and customs of the Old World, as an exciting venture into the new and unexplored. These colonists broke from the traditional restraints of their birthplace, and accepted change as welcome. We have seen that changes were desired, not only by adults, but children as well. The American Child Revolution brought to the young a kind of independence from parental controls, and particularly paternal authority, which wasn't dreamed of in the Old World.

The British anthropologist Geoffrey Gorer has commented upon this trait in the American character, the rejection of the father. In his book *The American People*,[17] he has reviewed the life of the early settlers who left England, and left with it the rule of the supreme father, the King. He points out that upon reaching this country they were careful to insure themselves against absolute rule in the future. They established a complicated system of checks and balances. The Executive was checked by the Legislative, the Legislative by the Judicial, and the Judicial by the individual Justices of the Supreme Court. To complete the circle, these Justices were to be appointed by the Executive on the approval of the Legislative.

Today we still see paternal rejection at work, in more concrete and dramatic terms. The emigrant is often unable to relinquish many of the customs and convictions of his fatherland. He hopes that his son will be a better American than he is. His ambition is that he will surpass him in education, in achievement, and in social status. Thus, his children are en-

313

couraged to break away from their family and start out early on their own.

Our country has very few large kinship groups. They survived almost to the present in the agricultural South, where families have subsisted on the products of their land. There are a few rather isolated groups of individuals who have come from other countries and cultures and have retained the traditions of their forebears. Such are the Chinese, as a whole still living apart in communities of their own, maintaining the close kinship of their own culture.

But with few exceptions Americans live in very small family groups. It was the custom of early settlers to go forth and seek a living where they could, and their children followed the pattern. In the early days it was land that beckoned the young man. Later, industry sprang up and he left his home to find a job wherever the opportunity might be. He would then take his wife and children with him, sometimes far from both families. America being a wide country, family visits often were made impossible. The airplane and the telephone now telescope distance, but, in the past, separation was almost complete. Then and now the husband and wife were on their own, making their own decisions, attempting to solve their own problems as they arose. Independence and self-reliance were the new demands.

The family is without roots today. Husband and wife are dependent upon one another, for they have no one else. Children must receive all family support from their parents. This could have made for close bonds. But in fact, it taxes each individual to a maximum level of maturity and strength. The family has grown smaller, and the need for stability and solidity of its members has taken on importance in proportion. The responsibility that was once diffused now rests almost entirely on two people, husband and wife.

It may be argued that much of the emotional sustenance and guidance of children today falls on such organizations as the school, the church, or, unfortunately, in some cases the courts. But until school age the child comes into very little contact with any of these outside of his parents. The start for emotional growth must then be entirely on them for a long time to come. The school and the church can only be complements, not substitutes for the parents.

Marriage, then, has a unique importance today. To the Roman individual the family was all, and depended entirely upon the father's power. The individual today depends on the family, which is now the partnership of two individuals. With the internal values at variance, the significance of the family to the social structure is very much the same. Nothing can be more important to society than the family. The family today rests precariously upon the individual and his preparedness for the role he is to play in it. Rather than on economic security, it is based on that particular form of enchanted blindness called Romantic Love. Romantic love may lead in any direction: to a strong and stable relation between two people, or just as easily to a neurotic relationship which will spell disaster to all emotionally involved.

The latter is far too often the case. From divorce statistics and psychiatric practice we know that many are the people who have married to satisfy a neurotic need—the need to dominate, to be dominated, to escape from parents, to find substitute parents, etc., needs which are not recognized as such, since they express unconscious desires. But, perhaps more unfortunate than these marriages ending in divorce are those which never reach the courts, the marriages in which so much hostility festers, yet the neurotic need of both partners is so intense that they cannot tear apart. A happy family life demands maturity. There is no maturity in these neurotic relations. The children who should gain emotional strength from their parents become heir, instead, to emotional ills. This is not a problem affecting individuals only. It affects every one of us, for it affects society. Only a strong family can provide individuals with the ego strength to live in confusing times. We have seen that the lack of discipline during the early years, often misinterpreted as an offering for self-expression, leads to weakness of the core of the personality. Self-expression and the acceptance of discipline are not incompatible. Indeed, the ultimate goal is freedom of the individual through self-discipline, since a man is not free who is a slave to his instinctual urges and the prey of outside influences, however tenuous or contradictory they may be. For a large part, ego strength and freedom of the individual rest upon self-discipline.

Those parents, unable to give early to their children the internal strength which will arm them against later frustrations, will have shown the same weakness prior to becoming parents. Many stories could be told of marriages made for misidentified reasons, and of the havoc these marriages played on the children and the children's children. Youngsters from these families make up the greatest number of young patients seen by psychiatrists. It is from the stories of three such children and their families that I shall give the briefest account to illustrate what happens when marriage is entered for these misidentified reasons.

The need to be tyrannically dominated cannot be a sound basis for the choice of a husband. And, yet, it may be the actual reason for some women to marry. It is the need that has made popular the tough men of stage and screen. It has brought success to such idols as Humphrey Bogart and Marlon Brando. But Hollywood passes over the subtler shadings and interreactions of these personalities. Presented in a marriage partnership, the man's neurotic need to dominate is relegated to obscurity, an obscurity wherefrom the perceptive movie-goer may or may not be able to retrieve it. But we must not forget that his wife has an equally neurotic need, the need to be dominated and to suffer. Each gets dubious gains from the marriage.

Peter Randolph is one of many such cruel and hostile husbands. His undeniable charm and intelligence easily concealed the violence of his nature. But both attracted at least one girl, Shirley. She admired his "masculine" aggressiveness, the appearance of a strength on which she could depend. She soon found out that even as a passive, obedient wife she could not stave off his bursts of temper or satisfy his demands, immaturity showing through.

And their child? His birth was a blow to the father's supremacy, a rival for the mother's attention. Peter's fits of temper grew more frequent and they were often directed at his child. No sooner was Robert brought home from the hospital than the quarrels began. The baby grew up hearing angry shouts. In his defense, and only then, did the mother dare oppose her husband. There were many hysterical scenes in response to angry threats.

When she dressed the child to go outdoors, Peter accused her of pampering him, of making a sissy of him. Did he himself need all the bundling up? When the baby had colds, the father snapped at her to stop fussing. It was the best way to make a weakling out of him. Sometimes Robert cried during dinner. The tension became unbearable. Then would Peter burst angrily at his wife, "Can't you make the brat shut up for a minute!" (To banish this competitor!)

As he grew older, the boy became conscious of the discord, taking it as his own responsibility. In a way which he could not analyze, it was. His father's rejection he perceived in every criticism, however small, his father levelled at him. His short life was to him a long failure. Once, as he lay awake in the dark hearing the quarrels in the next room, he heard his mother sobbing, "I wish I had never had the child!" At the age of eleven Robert was fortuitously saved from an attempt at suicide.

In its grim essentials this story is not overstated. It can hardly be said to be unique. The man glimpsed at has existed in every century. He has made many families miserable. In the patriarchal structure of the last century he might have been more in type, for he stood out then, as now, from the men around him. There is a difference. Was it then necessary for a man to bully in order to be master of his family? He might love his wife and children, offer them tenderness and consideration, but this could not weaken his position. He did not have to prove himself the "boss." That he was without challenge. The issues were not clouded by distribution of authority.

Mary's family life is far different from Robert's. But she is no happier. The roles of her parents are reversed. It is her mother who is the forceful, dominating partner, her father who plays the submissive role. Mary is sadly out of place in her family, the one person who doesn't feel she belongs. Her mother is a charming woman, involved in many social activities, the envy of women, the idol of men. Her clothes, her home, her possessions, are all beautiful. And one of her most handsome possessions is her husband, Mary's father, all-

American athlete, captain of his football team in college, outstanding on the polo field, and a successful business man, in addition. A man whose facile success with ladies of his set makes a wife at once pleased and a little uneasy.

Alma Davis has gone through a rapid succession of marriages, this being her third. To understand her today it is necessary to visualize her, however fleetingly, as a child. No sibling. Her mother left the home when she was barely six, and from then on she was left in charge of nurses, who were fired at varying rates of speed, depending on the child's whim. In the eyes of her father, who doted on her, she could do no wrong. If she said that Miss Smith, current nurse and ready target, was too strict, Miss Smith was not given a hearing. Out she went. Then Miss Smith's successor, who was really tough, went out even faster. "A spoiled child" was the estimation of those in the family who knew her earlier. More to the point, she was a child who never had to face frustrations, outside of the absence of frustrations.

The death of her father in her early twenties threw her into a mild depression. The depression is understandable, if you consider that she was so close to her father, part of him, and had very little inner strength to go on without him. Could she under her early life circumstances grow into a mature adult? She recovered without treatment, and it was not long after that that she married a man nearly twice her age. She divorced him fairly soon. Then a second marriage, not the happier for the smaller discrepancy in age. It seemed that with her third husband she had found some stability. She was then in her early thirties, a radiant creature, slightly hypomanic and scintillating in her conversation, some exhibitionism (with charm) in her manner, an index of her arrested emotional growth.

The search for the lost father appeared to have ended, and she was sure to have found "permanent love" at last. Her third marriage was to Rodman, then a tenacious suitor, the one among others who could convince her that he was unable to live without her. His courtship was a lavishing of attention, thoughtfulness, and other signs of love which tipped the scales. When they returned home from her third honeymoon, their happiness seemed complete. That is, until Mary was born.

It was at this time that the father became involved in his first infidelity, a casual affair, but one which was to be the first step in a long series. The baby had interrupted the carefree life of this couple. Alma had determined to give her child the love and affection she had felt deprived of. This she could give only in spurts. The romance was over. A child had no place in the existence of these two narcissistic people. Mary could serve as little but an attractive plaything for her mother. She did not arouse much interest in her father.

The baby grew up into a moody and dull-appearing little girl. She didn't fulfill her mother's hopes for a beautiful, golden-haired plaything, another possession to show off. Quite the contrary, she seemed intent on making herself as sparkless and inconspicuous as possible. She developed what her parents called "bad habits," pitting one parent against the other, lying her way out of trouble, and even "snitching."

Mary's father indulged more and more frequently in short-lived affairs. Always he came back to his wife. And always he was forgiven. It is easy to project one's conflicts onto others. Mary, they concluded, was the cause of their unhappiness. It was because of Mary that their marriage was floundering. Official reason given: the mobility of parental homes, as, indeed, these were young people who were ceaselessly seeking new horizons. Mary should have some permanence, if not of feelings, at least of surroundings. And so, Mary was at first sent away to "visit" a former governess. With her, after a short period of loneliness, she seemed for a period to flourish. She became more communicative and spontaneous, sought friends, and for the first time even did very good work at school.

At home, in the course of shorter and shorter visits, she was the child who tries hard to gain attention and win love by doing the very things that will invariably bring hostility and resentment in return. Gawky and blocked in her movements, she would attempt to climb on her father's lap, tug at her mother's sleeve, and interject herself into her parents' conversation. More and more annoyed and bewildered by her daughter's behavior, the mother came to refer to the child as "her cross to bear."

Unable to make a place in her own home, she was sent to a boarding school, a solution sought out for many a limp parent-child relationship. This was the final blow for Mary. Now there was no doubt left in her mind that her parents did not want her. Movie magazines and gorging of sweets became her favorite and all-absorbing pastimes. There is satisfaction and vicarious security in these. Food cravings substitute for love cravings. She now completely felt that she had failed her parents. No incentive, no interests. She is the unhappy victim of a neurotic marriage.

Emotional maladjustment is passed on from generation to generation. It may end when some outside influence appears to break the cycle, professional help, competent advice from church or social worker, or adequate parent substitution. In the story of the next family the cycle has remained unbroken for three generations. It may continue for a fourth.

The story was first told by Cynthia Rogers, a pretty woman, a bit too brightly dressed, just a little too conspicuously made-up. She came to the court of domestic relations with this to say. Her husband's lawyers had communicated with her and were threatening to withdraw her alimony, if she did not relinquish her children to her husband's family, a procedure not legally acceptable, but effective enough in its threatening overtones.

One child accompanied her to the office, a somewhat subdued, quiet little boy. While his mother talked, he played on the other side of the room with a small toy, seemingly absorbed in the activity. He was about four years old, the child left at home was a girl of six.

Her husband's family were "no good," she voiced rather heatedly. They had objected to her marrying him, because they were rich, "but their family is nothing to boast about," she continued. "Their daughter is a drunk and their granddaughter is away in a school for delinquent children. What right do they have to think that they alone are fit to have the children?" she asked. Her husband had no interest in them and it was their grandmother who really wanted them. Strange language from a woman who appeared gentle and unaggressive.

She told how her marriage had failed, projecting all responsibilities outside. Her husband, always a playboy, had almost immediately started going out with other women. Even during her first pregnancy he had been unfaithful to her. It was only for the children's sake, she added, that she had lasted with him as long as four years. It was finally her husband who had asked for the divorce, offering a generous settlement and willing to give the children up to her care. From that time on she had made every effort and had nothing to do with his family.

What about her children? it was asked. Were they happy without their father? The mother pointed to the younger child in the corner of the room—he was happy, easygoing, and complying. The other one, the girl, "took after her father's side of the family." She was at a loss in dealing with her.

The story was told a second time, this time by the paternal grandfather of the children in question. He was a distinguished-looking gentleman, a scholar by affinity and compulsion. He had retired to the world of books, partly as a solace for the frustrations in his married life. He had been reluctant to come to the interview, expressing his wish that the matter be dealt with through his lawyers.

The psychiatrist had insisted on seeing something of the paternal side. The grandfather had turned up unexpectedly. Reluctant, he was not uncommunicative. Family matters he discussed with a minimum of details. He explained first that he was coming instead of his son, who was away on a fishing trip.

The gist of his story was that "that woman" wasn't fit to bring up his grandchildren. As the words "that woman" came out, they seemed borrowed from another's vocabulary. His own style was too polished to admit of the epithet. His son had made an unfortunate marriage, but that was "all over now," and his wife was very anxious that the children be taken away from the bad influence of their mother as soon as possible. The little girl, in particular, was already showing how bad her influence could be. The probing did not allow bypassing of his own daughter. He mentioned very briefly that she had had a little trouble, yes, a nervous breakdown. Her child was away at boarding school, he volunteered. The school he named was very well known for offering psychiatric therapy to emotionally disturbed children.

Mr. Rogers' reserve was shunted aside as the interview neared a close. An initial interview often has this releasing effect. He offered to the psychiatrist, almost with relief, the information that his greatest concern was for his wife. She was very worried about the children and determined on getting them away from their mother. It is at this point that he added his most revealing comment. "I suppose that you would call my wife a typical 'Mom.' Our son would have made a better girl, our daughter a better boy." He would not elaborate further, but his meaning was clear.

We would not need to meet the grandmother in this family to know that her personality is at the root of her grandchildren's problems. She is familiar to us in many stories of divorce, in many unhappy homes. She is the mother of the emasculated boy, of the masculine girl. She is the domineering woman who longs to be a man. Considered as an individual, she is, nevertheless, in its group form the extreme of what woman's "emancipation" has led to.

Like many others of her kind, this woman intuitively sought out a passive man to marry. When her son was born, she transferred onto him what she was unable to give her husband. Through her son, she lived the male life she unconsciously craved. This son never had a chance to grow up as a man. His father, anyway, was a poor image to emulate. He too was unable to escape the mother-wife domination. Marriage, for this young father, did not mean self-assertion. He was emotionally unable to meet the responsibilities of a family. Indeed, at the moment of the interview, when he should have been concerned about the welfare of his children, he was off on a fishing trip.

His sister suffered too as a result of their domineering mother. From childhood on she was rejected in favor of her brother. The jealousy she felt could not be voiced, and she turned to her father for companionship, as one exile turns to another. Just as her brother could not escape identifying completely with his mother, so did she identify with her father.

322

Thus was her femaleness thwarted. Little wonder is it that she attempted to escape from this topsy-turvy family at the first opportunity. Her marriage was doomed to failure. The child, later conceived to hold it together, merely became part of the unhappy tangle.

Three generations are involved in this family tragedy. Two generations of children have paid the price. One granddaughter is under psychiatric care; the other is obviously disturbed. Only the little boy seems, at present, to have remained untroubled by his father's absence. At present, and on very superficial appraisal, he may escape the destructive influence of this family, although clinical experience would speak against it.

This story can be told again and again. The names may change, but the people are alike. Our age has, if not produced, at least accentuated the domineering woman, the "emancipated" woman who has the drive to live a man's life. This woman figures as the center of the drama. She emasculates her husband and weakens her children. Her relation to her son is a morbid one. His feelings remain confused on how much man, how much woman he is, on what role he must play. And so it is with the daughter. The pattern will be passed on from mother to child, from father to child, with its intricacies of neurotic dovetailing. How much can be undone? The facts and figures behind the general emotional maladjustment of our day have been quoted at intervals. They give very tangible answers.

The three stories were selected out of a large number of possibilities for their chiaroscuro effects and their reflection of great human misery. Not all emotional ills of one generation are passed on to the next with the impact we have found in these stories. By the same token, healthy emotional attitudes arising out of sound families are passed on along successive generations.

Obviously it is not enough to trace the conflicts back to their causes, in part woman's break from her earlier "feminine" position and her attempt to reach a footing equal with men. Historical knowledge may help clarify issues; it cannot solve them. Only the individual woman can do that. Taking stock of herself, recognizing her own dilemma, she can hope to work constructively in a direction which leads to readjustment and reintegration of those in the family unit.

Books, helpful as they are, are not the solution. If they were, we should see today enrichment rather than impoverishment of family life. Why is it that the family today must count on so many external and vicarious sources of "communication?" Why is it that modern man seems to be so easily prey to his anxiety? Why is it that he must seek panacea to his unrest in sources outside of himself and his own family? Television, for instance, has divided further rather than consolidated the family unit. Most entertainments have lost their spontaneity; they have taken on a routine and mechanical pattern which stunts individual expression and communication. This absence of knowledge of one another, this lack of closeness, is clearly reflected, for instance, in the lamentation of many a parent of teen-agers. Bewildered by some current behavior of their own teen-agers, they bewail, "I don't understand adolescents!" overlooking the fact that their one child, while being of a large group described as adolescents, remains their own particular child who has grown with them year after year. Somehow they have lost the thread of communication.

Without communication healthy discipline is difficult to apply and self-discipline difficult to acquire. Teen-agers, who will tomorrow have their own families, are now aware of the emotional gap between themselves and their parents. As acting Head of the United States Children's Bureau, Mrs. Elizabeth Ross referred to a group of teen-agers who had been able concisely to comment on the conflicts between the two generations. Two particular comments are worth noting. "Parents," they say, "are just about as hard to live with when they are too lenient as when they are too strict—anyway, they should be consistent. . . . Grown-ups spend years keeping children busy with made-up things to do to keep them out of mischief, and then expect adolescents suddenly to develop wholesome interests for themselves." Mrs. Ross pointed out that they were making significant observations in clearer terms than the Bureau was able to do after years of study.

Many a family today is a family in name only. Dealing at the periphery with its everyday arising problems may give a sense of immediate accomplishment. But does it reach the core? Only when parents will have regained a deep sense of the importance of their respective and well-defined role in fostering the emotional growth of their children, will they return the family to its ideal function in society.

POSTSCRIPT

Throughout this book I have raised more questions than given answers. Generally speaking, it can be said that in attempting to get the answers we must look at the family in which the disturbed child has been raised. We know that it takes mature parents to foster normal emotional growth. We have seen that not all marriages are the realization of a sound emotional relationship between two mature individuals. In telling numbers they are entered to satisfy immature, neurotic needs. Too often, those who are the core of the family, husband and wife, are, in effect, themselves children, victims of their parents' own mismotivated marriages.

A union of two people can be no more stable than the individuals entering this union. The individual of whom we talk a great deal is not as strong as we would have him. The pattern of the family has been altered in a few generations. Does it afford the strengthening each growing individual is assumed to receive from it? In a confusing crosscurrent of ideas and values man tends to vacillate and fails to develop the inner strength which he needs before disturbing realities.

Unsureness of self marks the individual of today. The woman is unsure of herself as a woman, the man of his role as a man. Compensations there are in the ersatz and machine-made satisfactions of our modern world. But do they make up for the inner void?

326

Nowhere is this more clearly reflected than in the attitude toward the child in the family today. It is a curiously detached attitude. The child has become "abstracted." He is not neglected. Far from it. There is an ever-increasing flow of information on the child reaching the general public. Lectures and discussion groups are available to the parent. "The Book" will provide an indexed guide to the youngster's daily needs, be it "freedom of expression," "balanced diet" or "discipline."

What more can the child need? A great deal—his parents' love and understanding, their closeness and support. Discipline is then not a thing apart. It is a complex and all-pervading reaching out to the child, who actually does not have a sense of being "disciplined." This insight cannot be found within the pages of a book. If it were the privilege of a book-acquired knowledge, would we find it in the unsophisticated type of parent such as Benjie's mother in *Children of Divorce?*

Ours is a generation and a country rich in substitutes. There is always an easy way out. Do we fail at times to see where it leads? Have we not made a fetish of easy living? The easy way in child care is usually over-indulgence, or unrelenting discipline, or sometimes both in alternation. Avowedly, the goal is not the child's emotional growth, it is rather the child's happiness—anything to put off the awful day of "growing-up." Only indulgence could save him from frustrations, a happy formula toward full contentment. Restraint cannot fail to become a necessity when the child becomes unmanageable. The fatal day must come when he will be "on his own." At that time, and often before, does the emotionally disturbed child make himself known.

Where does the explanation lie to our confusion and uncertainty in dealing with the child today? Has it perhaps its roots in those centuries of neglect and abuse of the child? Are we today feeling guilt over the long-forgotten child? A great upheaval came about, in large part through the American Child Revolution. The structure of the family and of society was deeply shaken. Confusion might well result in the too rapid changes that took place.

The answer to our confusion lies with every individual. Many problems have arisen from this confusion. We could attack them one by one, and so we do: juvenile delinquency, inadequacies of educational methods, divorce, and many others. The periphery, not the core. It is important that we take stock of ourselves, that we recognize the problem for what it is —weakened individuals and impoverished human relations.

Some constructive steps need to be taken to restore individual communication, to bring back unity in the family. There is danger that the parents of this generation will pass on their uncertainty to the next.

The problem is not the concern only of individuals. It affects society as a whole. Society is no stronger than the individuals who make it up. The children living today need the chance for a sound emotional development, if they are to have a sound family life of their own in the years to come. Only the stability and richness of family life can make strong individuals in the society of future generations.

NOTES AND REFERENCES

INTRODUCTION

1. Auden, W. H., *The Age of Anxiety: A Baroque Eclogue* (Faber and Faber, 1949).
2. May, R., *Man's Search for Himself* (W. W. Norton, 1953).
3. Tillich, P., *The Courage to Be* (Yale University Press, 1953).
4. Pennell, M. Y., Cameron, D., and Kramer, M., Mental Health Clinic Services for Children in the United States— 1950, *Public Health Reports, 66:* 1519, 1951.
5. Morse, W. W., and Limburg, C. C., "Availability and Use of Psychiatric Clinics, 1947," *Mental Health Statistics,* 1950.
6. Kanner, L., "The Origins and Growth of Child Psychiatry." *Am. J. Psych., 100:* 139, 1944.

PART ONE

1. Despert, J. L., *Children of Divorce* (Doubleday, 1953).

PART TWO. THE LONG-FORGOTTEN CHILD

1. Blumgart, L., "Observations on Maladjusted Children." *Mental Hygiene, 5:* 322, 1921.
2. Hazen, H. H., and Whitmore, E. R., "Skin Diseases Due to Emotional Disturbances." *Arch. Derm. and Syphil. 12:* 261, 1925.
3. Sullivan, E. B., "Emotional Disturbances Among Children." *Jour. Juv. Res., 16:* 56, 1932.
4. Menninger, W. C., "The Mentally and Emotionally Handicapped Veteran." *Ann. Amer. Acad. Pol. and Soc. Sci., 239:* 20, 1945.
5. Kanner, *op. cit.*

6. Zilboorg, G., and Henry, G. W., *A History of Medical Psychology* (W. W. Norton, 1941).

7. Since the writing of this book, there has appeared a work by Philippe Ariès, *L'Enfant et la Vie Familiale Sous L'Ancien Régime* (Librairie Plon, 1960), in which the emergence of family life and the role of the child is traced from the Middle Ages to the eighteenth century. But even in this scholarly study of contemporary chronicles, little information is obtained regarding the emotional aspects of children's lives during this period.

8. Le Grand D'Aussy, *Historie de la Vie Privée des Français* (Paris, 1782).

9. From Castigliano, A., *A History of Medicine,* trans. E. B. Krumbhaar (Knopf, 1941).

10. Lewis, W. H., *The Splendid Century* (Doubleday, 1957).

11. *The Holy Bible.* Authorized (King James) Version, Genesis XXI. 10.

12. Matthew II. 16.

13. II Kings XXII. 1.

14. *Ibid.*

15. Luke II. 40-52.

16. Daniel I. 2-4.

17. Drazin, N., *History of Jewish Education from 515 B.C.E. to 220 B.C.E. to 220 C.E.* University Studies in Education No. 29 (Johns Hopkins Press, 1940).

18. Graves, F. P., *A History of Education. Part one: Before the Middle Ages* (Macmillan, 1923).

19. Cubberly, E. P., *The History of Education* (Houghton Mifflin, 1920).

20. Cubberly, *op. cit.,* and Graves, *op. cit.*

21. Goodsell, W., *A History of Marriage and the Family* (Macmillan, 1934).

22. Cubberly, *op. cit.*

23. Graves, *op. cit.*

24. Klein, A. E., *Child Life in Greek Art* (Columbia University Press, 1932).

25. Graves, *op. cit.*

26. *Ibid.*

27. Goodsell, *op. cit.*

28. *Ibid.*

29. Beauvallet, R., *Etude Historique sur la Patria Potestas Considérée sur la Personne et les Biens de l'Enfant* (A. Davy, 1908).

30. Cicero (106-43 B.C.), *Pro Cecina.*

31. Thwing, C. F., and Thwing, C. B., *The Family: an Historical and Social Study* (Lee and Shepard, 1887).
32. Beauvallet, *op. cit.*
33. Goodsell, *op. cit.*
34. Graves, *op. cit.*
35. *Ibid.*
36. Quintilian, quoted by Goodsell, *op. cit.*
37. St. Augustin, *Les Confessions* (*Traduction nouvelle sur l'édition latine,* 1696).
38. Dill, S., *Roman Society in Gaul in the Merovingian Age* (Macmillan, 1926).
39. Thwing and Thwing, *op. cit.*
40. *Ibid.*
41. St. Bernardino, quoted in C. G. Coulton, *Life in the Middle Ages* (Cambridge University Press, 1921).
42. Zilboorg and Henry, *op. cit.*
43. Stuart, D. M., *The Girl Through the Ages* (Lippincott, 1933).
44. Coulton, *op. cit.*
45. *Ibid.*
46. Mackay, D. L., *Les Hôpitaux et la Charité à Paris au XIIIᵉ Siècle* (Honoré Champion, 1928).
47. Bonzon, J., *Cent Ans de Lutte Sociale: La Législation de L'Enfant 1789-1894* (Guillaumin, 1894).
48. Bercovici, K., *The Crusades* (Cosmopolitan Book Corp., 1929).
49. Runciman, S., *A History of the Crusades. Vol. III* (Cambridge University Press, 1954).
50. *Ibid.*
51. Bercovici, *op. cit.*
52. *Ibid.*
53. Zilboorg and Henry, *op. cit.*
54. Murray, M., *The God of the Witches* (Oxford University Press, 1952).
55. Murray, M., *Witch-Cult in Western Europe* (Clarendon Press, 1921).
56. Murray, *The God of the Witches.*
57. Murray, *Witch-Cult in Western Europe.*
58. Hastings, P., *Famous and Infamous Cases* (Roy Publishers, 1954).
59. Coulton, *op. cit.*
60. Murray, *The God of the Witches.*
61. Zilboorg and Henry, *op. cit.*
62. *Ibid.*
63. *Ibid.*

64. Mackay, *op. cit.*
65. Bonzon, *op. cit.*
66. Ribble, M. A., *The Rights of Infants* (Columbia University Press, 1943).
    ————, *The Personality of the Young Child* (Columbia University Press, 1955).
67. Spitz, R. A., and Wolf, K. M., "Anaclitic Depression," in *The Psychoanalytic Study of the Child*, Vol. II (International Universities Press, 1946).
68. Montaigne, *Les Essais, Nouvelle Edition* (Paris, 1725).
69. Burkhardt, J., *The Civilization of the Renaissance in Italy*, transl. S. G. C. Middlemore (Macmillan, 1928).
70. *Ibid.*
71. Jerrold, M. F., *Italy in the Renaissance* (Methuen, 1927).
72. *Ibid.*
73. Burkhardt, *op. cit.*, and Jerrold, *op. cit.*
74. Jerrold, *op. cit.*
75. Burkhardt, *op. cit.*
76. Low, A. M., *The Past Presented* (Peter Davies, 1952).
77. *Ibid.*
78. Murray, *Witch-Cult in Western Europe*.
79. *Ibid.*
80. *Ibid.*
81. Montaigne, *op. cit.*
82. Zilboorg and Henry, *op. cit.*
83. *Ibid.*
84. *Ibid.*
85. *Ibid.*
86. Calhoun, A. W., *A Social History of the American Family from Colonial Times to the Present* (Barnes and Noble, 1945).
87. *Ibid.*
88. *Ibid.*
89. *Ibid.*
90. *Ibid.*
91. *Ibid.*
92. *Ibid.*
93. Huxley, A., *The Devils of Loudun* (Harper and Bros., 1952).
94. Lewis, *op. cit.*
95. Taine, H. A., *The Ancient Regime*, transl. J. Durand (Henry Holt and Co., 1896).
96. Lewis, *op. cit.*
97. Murray, *Witch-Cult in Western Europe*.

98. Mitchell, R. J., *A History of the English People* (Longmans, Green and Co., 1950).

99. Gwyther, J., *First Voyage* (Andrew Melrose, 1954).

100. Mitchell, *op. cit.*

101. *Ibid.*

102. *Ibid.*

103. *Ibid.*

104. *Ibid.*

105. De La Mare, W., *Early One Morning* (Macmillan, 1935).

106. Mitchell, *op. cit.*

107. De La Mare, *op. cit.*

108. Mitchell, *op. cit.*

109. Murray, *Witch-Cult in Western Europe.*

110. Mitchell, *op. cit.*

111. Duval, L., *L'Etat Moral des Populations Agricoles au XVIIIᵉ Siècle dans la Généralité d'Alençon: Essais Tentés à Cette Epoque pour Fixer les Enfants Assistés à la Campagne* (Alençon, 1913).

112. *Ibid.*

113. Bonzon, *op. cit.* (My transl.)

114. *Ibid.*

115. *Ibid.*

116. Taine, *op. cit.*

117. Bonzon, *op. cit.*

118. Rousseau, J. J., *Emile or Concerning Education,* transl. E. Worthington (D.C. Heath and Co., 1888).

119. *Ibid.*

120. *Ibid.*

121. *Ibid.*

122. *Ibid.*

123. *Ibid.*

124. *Ibid.*

125. *Ibid.*

126. *Ibid.*

127. Ashton, J., *Social Life in the Reign of Queen Anne* (Chatto and Windus, 1929).

128. Quoted by Mitchell, *op. cit.*

129. *Ibid.*

130. Ashton, *op. cit.*

131. Young, *My Forty Years at the Yard* (W. H. Allen, 1955).

132. Hastings, *op. cit.*

133. Mitchell, *op. cit.*

134. De La Mare, *op. cit.*

135. *Ibid.*

136. Griffiths, A., *The Chronicles of Newgate, Vol. II* (Chapman Hall, 1884).

137. *Ibid.*

138. Wilde, O., *Children in Prison and Other Cruelties of Prison Life* (Pamphlet—a letter to the Editor of the *Daily Chronicle*, London, 1898).

139. *Ibid.*

140. *Ibid.*

141. Griffiths, *op. cit.*

142. Barnes, H. E., *The Story of Punishment* (Stratford, 1930).

143. Mitchell, *op. cit.*

144. Guerard, A. L., *French Civilization in the Nineteenth Century* (The Century Co., 1914).

145. Tyson, H. G., "Day Nursery" in *Encyclopaedia of the Social Sciences*, Vol. 5 (Macmillan, 1937).

146. Edwards, B., *Home Life in France* (McClung and Co., 1905).

147. Depitre and Levique, *La Réduction du Nombre des Enfants Employés la Nuit dans les Verreries*. Part 2 (Paris, 1911).

148. Barker, E. H., *France of the French* (Scribner's, 1909).

149. Edwards, *op. cit.*

150. Klein, P., "Delinquent Children" in *Encyclopaedia of the Social Sciences*, Vol. 3 (Macmillan, 1937).

151. Bonzon, *op. cit.*

152. Calhoun, *op. cit.*

153. *Ibid.*

154. *Ibid.*

155. *Ibid.*

156. *Ibid.*

157. *Ibid.*

158. *Ibid.*

159. *Ibid.*

160. Barnes, *op. cit.*

PART THREE. THE EMOTIONALLY HEALTHY CHILD

1. Menninger, K. A., *The Human Mind* (Knopf, 1955).

2. Binger, C., *More About Psychiatry* (University of Chicago Press, 1949).

3. Mead, M., *New Lives for Old* (Morrow, 1956).

4. Kanner, L., *Child Psychiatry* (Charles C. Thomas, 1935).

5. Hamilton, A. E., *Emotional Aspects of Pregnancy* (Ph.D. Dissertation, Columbia University, 1955).

6. Monakow, C. V., and Mourgue, R., *Introduction Biologique à l'Etude de la Neurologie et Psychopathologie* (Alcan, 1928).

7. Freud, S., *New Introductory Lectures on Psychoanalysis*. Transl. W. S. H. Sprott (W. W. Norton, 1933).

8. Rank, O., *The Trauma of Birth* (Harcourt, Brace and Co., 1929).

9. Despert, J. L., "Anxiety, Phobias and Fears in Young Children—with Special Reference to Prenatal, Natal and Neonatal Factors." *Nervous Child, 5:* 8, 1946.

10. Greenacre, P., "The Biological Economy of Birth" in *The Psychoanalytic Study of the Child,* Vol. I (International Universities Press, 1945).

11. Levy, D., *Primary Affect Hunger. Am. J. Psych., 94:* 643, 1937.

12. Spitz, R., "Hospitalism: An Inquiry into the Genesis of Psychiatric Conditions in Early Childhood" in *The Psychoanalytic Study of the Child,* Vols. I and II (International Universities Press, 1945/1946).

13. Despert, J. L., "Urinary Control and Enuresis." *Psychosom. Med., 6:* 293, 1944.

14. Huschka, M., "A Study of Training in Voluntary Control of Urination in a Group of Problem Children." *Psychosom. Med., 5:* 254, 1943.

15. Despert, J. L., "Emotional Aspects of Speech and Language Development." *Monatssch. f. Psych. und Neurol., 104:* 193, 1941.

16. Halls, G. S., *Adolescence* (Appleton and Co., 1904).

17. Groos, K., *The Play of Man,* transl. E. L. Baldwin (Appleton and Co., 1919).

18. Despert, J. L., "A Method for the Study of Personality Reactions in Preschool Children by Means of Analysis of Their Play." *J. Psychol., 9:* 17, 1940.

19. Despert, J. L., "A Comparative Study of Thinking in Schizophrenic Children and Children of Preschool Age." *Am. J. Psych., 97:* 189, 1940.

20. Despert, J. L., "Dreams in Children of Preschool Age" in *The Psychoanalytic Study of the Child,* Vol. 3-4 (International Universities Press, 1949).

PART FOUR. THE EMOTIONALLY DISTURBED CHILD

1. Goldstein, K., *The Organism: A Holistic Approach to Biology Derived from Pathological Data in Man* (American Book Co., 1939).

2. Cannon, W. B., *The Wisdom of the Body* (W. W. Norton, 1932).

3. Freud, *op. cit.*

4. Rank, *op. cit.*

5. Adler, A., *The Individual Psychology of Alfred Adler,* ed. H. L. Ansbacher and R. R. Ansbacher (Basic Books, 1956).

335

6. Horney, K., *Neurosis and Human Growth: The Struggle Toward Self-Realization* (W. W. Norton, 1950).

7. Despert, *op. cit.*

8. Freud, *op. cit.*

9. *Ibid.*

10. *Ibid.*

11. *Ibid.*

12. *Ibid.*

13. *Ibid.*

14. Spitz, *Hospitalism*—I.

15. Spitz, *Hospitalism*—II.

16. Spitz and Wolf, *Anaclitic Depression.*

17. Spitz, R., "Anxiety in Infancy: A Study of Its Manifestations in the First Year of Life." *Int. J. Psychoanal., 31:* 138, 1950.

18. Goldfarb, W., "The Effect of Early Institution Care on the Adolescent Personality." *Child Development, 14:* 213, 1944.

19. Bowlby, E. J. M., *Maternal Care and Mental Health.* W. H. O. Monographs, #2, 1951.

20. Gelinier-Ortigues, and Aubry, J., "Maternal Deprivation, Psychogenic Deafness and Pseudo-Retardation" in *Emotional Problems of Early Childhood,* ed. G. Caplan (Basic Books, 1955).

21. Levesque, J., "*L'Anorexie du Nourrisson.*" *Bull. Med. 68:* 233, 1948.

22. Debre, R., and Mozziconacci, P., "*L'Anorexie Nerveuse de l'Enfant et le Problème de la Faim et de l'Appetit.*" *La Semaine des Hôpitaux de Paris, 26:* 454, 1954: "*Etude Psychosomatique de l'Anorexie Nerveuse,*" *ibid.,* 456.

23. Spitz, *Anaclitic Depression.*

24. Kanner, *Child Psychiatry.*

25. *Ibid.*

26. Levy, D. M., "Maternal Overprotection and Rejection." *Arch. Neurol. and Psych., 25:* 886, 1931.

27. Levy, *Primary Affect Hunger.*

28. *Ibid.*

29. *Ibid.*

30. Levy, *Maternal Overprotection.*

31. Despert, J. L., and Pierce, H. O., "The Relation of Emotional Adjustment to Intellectual Function." *Genet. Psychol. Monogr., 34:* 3, 1946.

32. These clinical cases and reports have been published in *Emotional Problems of Childhood,* ed. G. Caplan (Basic Books, 1955).

33. Kanner, L., "Autistic Disturbances of Affective Contact." *Nervous Child*, 2: 217, 1943.

34. Kanner, L., and Eisenberg, L., "Notes on the Follow-Up Study of Autistic Children" in *Psychopathology of Childhood*, ed. P. Hoch and J. Zubin (Grune and Stratton, 1955).

35. Kanner, L., "Problems of Nosology and Psychodynamics of Early Infantile Autism." *Am. J. Orthopsych.*, 19: 416, 1949.

36. Kanner, L., "Irrelevant and Metaphorical Language in Early Infantile Autism." *Am. J. Psych.*, 103: 242, 1946.

37. Kanner, *Problems of Nosology and Psychodynamics*.

38. Ssucharewa, G. E., "Uber den Verlauf der Schizophrenien in Kindersalters." *Zeitschr. für die gesamte Neurol. und Psychiat.*, 142: 309, 1932.

39. Grebelskaja-Albatz, E., "Zur Klinik der Schizophrenie des Fruhen Kindersalters." Schweiz. *Archiv. für Neurol. und Psych.*, 34: 244, 1934 and 35: 30, 1935.

40. Despert, J. L., "Schizophrenia in Children." *Psych. Quart.*, 12: 366, 1938. Revised from the address of July 26, 1937, at the First International Congress of Child Psychiatry, Paris, France.

41. Kanner, *Problems of Nosology and Psychodynamics*.

42. Kanner, L., "The Conception of Wholes and Parts in Early Infantile Autism." *Am. J. Psych.*, 108: 23, 1951.

43. Bleuler, E., *Dementia Praecox or the Group of Schizophrenias*, transl. J. Zinkin (International Universities Press, 1950).

44. Reprinted in full from Despert, J. L., "Some Considerations Relating to the Genesis of Autistic Behavior in Children." *Am. J. Orthopsych.*, 21: 335, 1951.

45. Peck, H., Rabinovitch, R. D., and Cramer, J. B., "A Treatment Program for Parents of Schizophrenic Children." *Am. J. Orthopsych.*, 19: 592, 1949.

46. Bender, L., "Childhood Schizophrenia." *Am. J. Orthopsych.*, 17: 40, 1947.

47. Despert, "Schizophrenia in Children."

48. Kanner, *Autistic Disturbances of Affective Contact*.

49. Tietze, T., "A Study of Mothers of Schizophrenic Patients." *Psychiatry*, 12: 55, 1949.

50. *Ibid.*

51. Kanner, *Autistic Disturbances of Affective Contact*.

52. Ribble, *op. cit.*

53. Spitz. See Notes 14, 15 and 16 above.

54. Kanner, *Problems of Nosology and Psychodynamics*.

55. Despert, J. L., "A Therapeutic Approach to the Problem of Stuttering in Children." *Nervous Child, 2:* 134, 1943.

56. Despert, J. L., "Stuttering: a Clinical Study." *Am. J. Orthopsych., 13:* 517, 1943.

57. Despert, J. L., "Psychopathology of Stuttering." *Am. J. Psych., 99:* 881, 1943.

58. Despert, J. L., "Psychosomatic Study of 50 Stuttering Children," *Am. J. Orthopsych., 16:* 100, 1946.

59. Despert, J. L., reprinted from "Psychopathology of Stuttering."

60. Dreikurs, R., "A Child with Compulsive Neurosis." *Indiv. Psychol. Bull., 6:* 137, 1947.

61. Despert, J. L., "Differential Diagnosis Between Obsessive-Compulsive Neurosis and Schizophrenia in Children" in *Psychopathology of Childhood,* ed. P. Hoch and J. Zubin (Grune and Stratton, 1955).

62. Goldfarb, W., and Dorsen, M. M., *Annotated Bibliography of Childhood Schizophrenia and Related Disorders* (Basic Books, 1956).

63. Bender, L. M., "Clinical Research on Schizophrenic Children Under Six" in *Emotional Problems of Early Childhood,* ed. G. Caplan (Basic Books, 1955).

64. Potter, H. W., "Schizophrenia in Children." *Am. J. Psych., 89:* 1253, 1933.

65. Ssucharewa, *op. cit.*

66. Grebelskaja-Albatz, *op. cit.*

67. Bender, L. M., "Behavior Problems in the Children of Psychotic and Criminal Parents." *Genet. Psychol. Monogr., 19:* 229, 1937.

68. Potter, *op. cit.*

69. Bender, L. M., "Childhood Schizophrenia." *Am. J. Orthopsych., 17:* 40, 1947.

70. Despert, "Schizophrenia in Children."

71. Mahler, M. S., "On Child Psychosis and Schizophrenia, Autistic and Symbiotic Infantile Psychoses" in *The Psychoanalytic Study of the Child,* Vol. 7 (International Universities Press, 1952).

72. Rank, B., Adaptation of the Psychoanalytic Technique for the Treatment of Young Children with Atypical Development. *Am. J. Orthopsych., 19:* 130, 1949.

73. Beres, D., and Obers, S.J., "The Effects of Extreme Deprivation in Infancy on Psychic Structure in Adolescence" in *The Psychoanalytic Study of the Child,* Vol. 5 (International Universities Press, 1950).

74. Despert, J. L., "Treatment in Child Schizophrenia" in *An Outline of Abnormal Psychology,* ed. Murphy and Bachrach (Modern Library, 1954).

75. Despert, J. L., Reprinted in part from "Differential Diagnosis Between Obsessive-Compulsive Neurosis and Schizophrenia in Children."

76. Alexander, F., "Der Neurotische der Character. Seine Steilung in der Psychopathologie und in der Literatur." *Int. Zeitsch. für Psychoanal., 14:* 26, 1928.

77. Hendrickson, R. C., *Youth in Danger* (Harcourt, Brace and Co., 1956).

78. Glueck, S., and Glueck, E., *One Thousand Juvenile Delinquents* (Harvard University Press, 1934).

79. Monroe, K., "A Better Way to Adopt a Baby." *Harper's Magazine,* January, 1957.

PART FIVE. REFLECTIONS ON THE FAMILY

1. Parsons, T., *The Family, Its Function and Destiny* (Harper and Bros., 1949).

2. Ribble, *op. cit.*

3. Despert, *op. cit.*

4. Gorer, G., *The American People: a Study in National Character* (W. W. Norton, 1948).

5. Despert, J. L., "Is Juvenile Delinquency a Psychiatric Problem?" *Nervous Child, 6:* 371, 1947.

6. Glueck, S. and Glueck, E., *One Thousand Juvenile Delinquents.*

7. Glueck, S. and Glueck, E., *Five Hundred Delinquent Women* (Knopf, 1934).

8. Strecker, E. A., *Their Mother's Sons* (Lippincott, 1946).

9. Wylie, P., *A Generation of Vipers* (Rinehart, 1955).

10. Orwell, G., *Such, Such Were the Joys* (Harcourt, Brace and Co., 1953).

11. Reported in *Family Life,* ed. P. Popenoe. IX, September, 1949.

12. Isaacs, S., *Social Development in Young Children* (Routledge, 1933).

13. English, O. S., *Bull. Menninger Clinic, 14:* 66, 1950.

14. Despert, *op. cit.*

15. Gorer, *op. cit.*

16. Despert, *op. cit.*

17. Gorer, *op. cit.*

ANCHOR BOOKS

PSYCHOLOGY